The Tarascon Internal Medicine & Critical Care Pocketbook

D1615658

You can find Tarascon books at your local medical bookstore, or order directly from Tarascon Publishing by sending a check to the address below (sorry, no credit cards). There is no extra charge for tax or shipping on most orders. Foreign orders must be prepaid in US dollars.

The Internal Medicine & Critical Care Pocketbook, 1st Edition
- $9.95 per copy, or $8.25 per copy for orders of 10 or more.

The Tarascon Pocket Pharmacopoeia, updated annually
- $6.95 per copy, or $5.75 per copy for orders of 10 or more.

The Pediatric Emergency Pocketbook, 2nd Edition
- $9.95 per copy, or $8.25 per copy for orders of 10 or more.

Tarascon Publishing, Box 1522, Loma Linda, California 92354

Important Caution - Please Read This!

The information in *Internal Medicine & Critical Care Pocketbook* is compiled from sources believed reliable. Despite exhaustive fact-checking efforts, this book may contain typographical errors and omissions. *Therefore we cannot guarantee the accuracy and completeness of this work.* The IMCCP is intended to be a quick and convenient reminder of information already learned elsewhere. Health care professionals should use sound clinical judgment and individualized therapy in each specific patient care situation. This book is not meant to be a replacement for training, experience, continuing medical education, or for studying the latest drug prescribing literature. Furthermore, not all therapy described here is endorsed by the US Food and Drug Administration. You are advised carefully to review package inserts before administering any medications. This book is sold without warranties of any kind, express or implied, and the publisher and editors disclaim any liability, loss, or damage caused by the contents. *If you do not wish to be bound by the foregoing cautions and conditions, you may return this book to the publisher for a full refund.*

Note from the author: The *IMCCP* is intended as a "head of the bed" reference for a variety of internal medicine emergencies. Early editions have been tested "in the trenches" by housestaff at University Hospitals of Cleveland and at University of California San Francisco; I am grateful for their input. If you find an error, **please** let me know; otherwise, a pox on you!

For brevity, I have included immediately life-threatening or less-common clinical problems (eg pituitary apoplexy) and omitted many common problems (eg diabetic ketoacidosis), for which most physicians need not consult a manual. To use this book effectively, please take a few minutes to familiarize yourself with its structure and contents.

I dedicate the *IMCCP* to John Leland Johnson, MD, a great doctor and a great teacher.

Artwork: *Examination of a Leper* by Hans von Gersdorff, Strasbourg, 1540. Courtesy of the National Library of Medicine, Images from the History of Medicine.

Robert J. Lederman, MD, Division of Cardiology, Department of Medicine, The University of Michigan Medical Center. rlederman@umich.edu.

Abbreviations

↓: decrease, low
↑: increase, high
∆: change
ABC: airway, breathing, circulation
ABG: arterial blood gas
AC: assist-control
ACh: acetylcholine
ACE: angiotensin converting enzyme
ACLS: Advanced cardiac life support
ADH: antidiuretic hormone
A-fib: atrial fibrillation
AI: aortic insufficiency
ALL: acute lymphoblastic leukemia
ALT: alanine aminotransferase
AML: acute myelogenous leukemia
Amp: ampule
ANA: antinuclear antibody
APTT: activated partial thromboplastin time
ARDS: adult respiratory distress syndrome
AS: aortic stenosis
ASD: atrial septal defect
AST: aspartate aminotransferase
ATN: acute tubular necrosis
AV: atrioventricular
AVB: atrioventricular block
AWMI: anterior wall myocardial infarction
BBB: bundle branch block
BMT: bone marrow transplant
BP: Blood pressure
Ca: calcium
CABG: coronary artery bypass graft
CAD: coronary artery disease
CAPD: continuous ambulatory peritoneal dialysis
CAVH/D: continuous arteriovenous hemofiltration/dialysis

CCS: Canadian cardiovascular society angina class
CHB: complete heart block
CHF: congestive heart failure
CL_{Cr}: creatinine clearance
CLL: chronic lymphocytic leukemia
CMV: cytomegalovirus
CN: cyanide
CNS: central nervous system
CO: carbon monoxide
COPD: chronic obstructive pulmonary disease
Cox: cyclooxygenase
CPK: creatine phosphokinase
CPR: cardiopulmonary resuscitation
Cr: creatinine
CR: complete remission
CRI: chronic renal insufficiency
CS: coronary sinus
CSF: cerebrospinal fluid
CT: computed tomography
CXR: chest radiograph
d: day
D5W: dextrose 5% in water
D50: dextrose 50% in water
DA: dopamine
DBA: dobutamine
DBP: diastolic BP
DI: diabetes insipidus
DIC: disseminated intravascular coagulation
DKA: diabetic ketoacidosis
dL: deciliter
d/o: disorder
DVT: deep vein thrombosis
DM: diabetes mellitus
DT: delirium tremens
Dz: disease
ECG: electrocardiogram
EEG: electroencephalogram
EMD: electromechanical dissociation
EP: electrophysiologic testing
Epi: epinephrine
ER: estrogen receptor

ESRD: end-stage renal disease
EtOH: ethanol
FDP: fibrin degradation products
FEV_1: forced expiratory volume in 1 second
F_1O_2: inspired oxygen fraction
FFP: fresh frozen plasma
FN: false negative
FP: false positive
FVC: forced vital capacity
G-6-PD: glucose-6-phosphatase deficiency
GFR: glomerular filtration rate
Glc: glucose
GI: gastrointestinal
gm: gram
GPC: gram-positive cocci
GNR: gram-negative rod
gtt: infusion
GVHD: graft versus host disease
h: hour
HA: headache
Hb: hemoglobin
HCM: hypertrophic cardiomyopathy
HCO_3^-: bicarbonate
H&P: history and physical exam
HR: heart rate
HSV: herpes simplex virus
HTN: hypertension
IABP: intraaortic balloon counterpulsation pump
IC_{50}: 50% inhibitory concentration
ICP: intracranial pressure
ICU: intensive care unit
IJ: internal jugular
IOP: intraocular pressure
IM: intramuscular
IU: international units
IV: intravenous
IVC: inferior vena cava
IVP: intravenous push
IWMI: inferior wall myocardial infarction

JVP: jugular vein pressure
K: potassium
L: left, liter
LA: left atrium
LAO: left anterior oblique
LAFB: left anterior fascicle block
LBBB: left bundle branch block
LDH: lactate dehydrogenase
LN: lymph node
LPFB: left posterior fascicle block
LV: left ventricle
LVEDP: left ventricular end-diastolic pressure
LVH: left ventricular hypertrophy
MAOI: monoamine oxidase inhibitor
MCTD: mixed connective tissue disease
MetHb: methemoglobin
mg: milligram
Mg: magnesium
MI: acute myocardial infarction
min: minutes
MIP: maximum inspiratory pressure
mL: milliliter
MS: mental status, multiple sclerosis, mitral stenosis
M_vO_2: myocardial oxygen consumption
MVV: maximum voluntary ventilation in 1 minute
MW: Molecular weight
Na: sodium
NE: norepinephrine
NHL: non-Hodgkin lymphoma
NIF: negative inspiratory force
NI: normal
NS: normal (0.9%) saline
NSAID: nonsteroidal antiinflammatory drug
NTG: nitroglycerin
N/V/D: nausea, vomiting, diarrhea

P: phosphorus
PA: pulmonary artery, posteroanterior
PAgram: pulmonary arteriogram
PCA: procainamide
P_aCO_2: partial pressure of carbon dioxide
PCP: *Pneumocystis carinii* pneumonia
PCWP: pulmonary capillary wedge pressure
PE: pulmonary thromboembolism
PEEP: positive end-expiratory pressure
PFT: pulmonary function test
po: orally
P_aO_2: arterial partial pressure of oxygen
P_AO_2: alveolar partial pressure of oxygen
PS: pressure support
PSVT: paroxysmal supraventricular tachycardia
Pt: patient
PT: prothrombin time
PTCA: percutaneous transluminal coronary angioplasty
PTX: pneumothorax
PUD: peptic ulcer disease
PVD: peripheral vascular disease
R: right
RA: right atrium
RAO: right anterior oblique
RBBB: right bundle branch block
RBC: red blood cell
RF: rheumatoid factor
RTA: renal tubular acidosis
RTX: radiation therapy
RV: right ventricle
Rx: therapy
SA: sinoatrial
SAH: subarachnoid hemorrhage
S_aO_2: arterial oxygen saturation

SBP: systolic BP
SIADH: syndrome of inappropriate ADH secretion
SIMV: intermittent mandatory ventilation
SLE: systemic lupus erythematosus
SQ: subcutaneous
SVC: superior vena cava
SVR: systemic vascular resistance
SVT: supraventricular tachycardia
T½: half-life
TB: tuberculosis
TCA: tricyclic antidepressant
TdP: Torsades de pointes
TIA: transient ischemic attack
Tid: three times daily
TBW: total body water
TCP: transcutaneous pacemaker
TEE: transesophageal echocardiography
TMP/SMX: trimethoprim-sulfamethoxazole
TN: true negative
TP: true positive
TPN: Total parenteral nutrition
TTP: thrombotic thrombocytopenia purpura
Tx: therapy
U: Unit
UAO: upper airway obstruction
UGI: upper gastrointestinal
U/S: ultrasound
VC: vital capacity
VF, V-Fib: ventricular fibrillation
V/Q: ventilation/perfusion
VSD: ventricular septal defect
VT, V-Tach: ventricular tachycardia
VZV: varicella-zoster virus
WBC: white blood cell
WPW: Wolff-Parkinson-White syndrome

Handy Formulas

Acid-Base Rules of Thumb[1]

Henderson-Hasselbach Equation

$$pH = pK + \log([HCO_3^-] / (0.03 \times pCO_2)); \quad [H] = 24 \times \frac{pCO_2}{HCO_3}(\times 10^{-7}\,M)$$

Acute Respiratory Acidosis (within 12-24 hrs)

↑: $\Delta[HCO_3^-] = (\Delta PaCO_2/10) \pm 3$

↓: $\Delta pH = .008 \times \uparrow\Delta PaCO_2$

Chronic Respiratory Acidosis $PaCO_2 = 2.4 \times [HCO_3^-] - 22$

↑: Δ plasma $[HCO_3^-] = .4 \times (\Delta PaCO_2)$ (± 4)

Acute Respiratory Alkalosis

↑: $\Delta pH = .008 \times \downarrow\Delta PaCO_2$

↓: $\Delta[HCO_3^-] = (.1\ to\ .3) \times (\Delta PaCO_2)$ (usually not to less than 18mM)

Chronic Respiratory Alkalosis

↓: $\Delta[HCO_3^-] = (.2\ to\ .5) \times (\Delta PaCO_2)$ (usually not to less than 18mM)

Metabolic Acidosis $PaCO_2 = 1.5 * [HCO_3^-] + 8$ (±2);

↓: $\Delta PaCO_2 = (1.0\ to\ 1.5) \times \Delta[HCO_3^-]$ $PaCO_2 \cong$ last two digits of pH

Metabolic Alkalosis $PaCO_2 = 0.9 * [HCO3-] + 9$ (±2)

↑: $\Delta PaCO2 = (0.25\ to\ 1.0) \times \Delta[HCO3-]$

---

pH	[H+]	pH	[H+]	pH	[H+]	pH	[H+]
6.90	125	7.12	76	7.34	46	7.58	27
6.92	120	7.14	73	7.36	44	7.60	25
6.94	115	7.16	70	7.38	42	7.62	24
6.96	110	7.18	66	7.40	40	7.64	23
6.98	105	7.20	63	7.44	37	7.66	22
7.00	100	7.22	60	7.46	35	7.68	21
7.02	95	7.24	58	7.48	33	7.70	20
7.04	91	7.26	55	7.50	32	7.72	19
7.06	87	7.28	52	7.52	30	7.74	18
7.08	83	7.30	50	7.54	29	7.76	17
7.10	80	7.32	48	7.56	28	7.78	17

---

[1] RW Schrier, <u>Renal and electrolyte disorders</u>, 3/e, Boston: Little-Brown, 1986.

Acid-Base Maps[2]

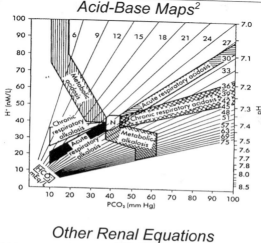

Other Renal Equations

$$\text{Calculated Osmolarity(mM)} = 2 \times Na(mM) + \frac{BUN(mg/dL)}{2.8} + \frac{Glucose(mg/dL)}{18} + \frac{EtOH(mg/dL)}{4.6}$$

(Normal 275 - 290 mOsm / kg)

$$\text{Osmolal Gap} = \text{Measured Osmolality} - \frac{\text{Calculated Osmolarity}}{0.93 \text{ (Serum 93\% water)}}$$ (Normal < 10 mOsm)

$$\text{Anion Gap} = [Na] - [Cl] - [HCO3]$$ (Normal 9 - 13 mmol / L)

$$\text{Creatinine Clearance} = \frac{Ucr \cdot V}{Pcr} = \frac{[\text{Urine creatinine (mg / dL)}] \cdot [\text{Urine volume (ml / Day)}]}{[\text{Plasma creatinine (mg / dL)}] \cdot 1440 \text{ min / Day}}$$

(Normal 75 - 160 ml / min)

$$\text{Creatinine Clearance} \approx \frac{140 - \text{Age (yrs)}}{\text{Serum Creatinine (mg / dL)} \times 72} \times \text{Weight (kg)} \ (\times 0.85 \text{ If Woman})$$

$$\text{Fractional Excretion of Sodium (FENa)} = \frac{[\text{Urine Na}] \times [\text{Plasma Cr}]}{[\text{Urine Cr}] \times [\text{Plasma Na}]}$$ (Prerenal azotemia < 0.01)

Potassium and pH: [K] increases 0.6 mEq / L for each pH drop of 0.1
Sodium and Glucose: [Na] depressed 1.6 mEq / L for each 100 mg / dL increase of Glucose
Calcium and Albumin: [Ca] decreases 0.8 mg / dL for each 1.0 gm / dL decrease in Albumin

---

[2] Goldberg M, et al, "Computer-based instruction and diagnosis of acid-base disorders," JAMA, 1973;223(3):269-75. Copyright 1973, American Medical Association, with permission.

Pharmacology Equations

Clearance: $\quad CL = V_d \times K_{el}$

Half-life: $\quad T_{1/2} = \dfrac{0.693}{K_{el}} = \dfrac{0.693 \times V_d}{CL}$

Elimination Constant $\quad K_{el} = \dfrac{\ln \dfrac{[peak]}{[trough]}}{Time_{peak} - Time_{trough}}$

Loading dose $\quad = V_d \times [target\ peak]$

Dosing interval $\quad = \dfrac{1}{K_{el}} \times \ln \dfrac{[desired\ peak]}{[desired\ trough]} + Infusion\ time$

Ideal Body Weight (Male) $= 50\ kg + (2.3\ kg\ per\ inch\ over\ 5\ feet)$

Ideal Body Weight (Female) $= 45\ kg + (2.3\ kg\ per\ inch\ over\ 5\ feet)$

Abbreviations: CL = clearance; V_d = Volume of distribution; K_{el} = elimination constant; $T\frac{1}{2}$ = Half-life; $\ln$ = natural (base e) logarithm

Hemodynamic Equations

Blood pressure: $\quad MAP = \dfrac{Systolic\ BP + (2 \times Diastolic\ BP)}{3} = DBP + \dfrac{SBP - DBP}{3}$

Fick Cardiac Output: $\quad CI = \dfrac{CO}{BSA} = (Normal\ 2.5 - 4.2\ L\,/\,min\,/\,m^2)$

$\quad CO = \dfrac{O_2\ Consumption}{(Arterial - Venous)\ O_2\ Content}$

$\quad CO = \dfrac{10 \times VO_2\ (ml\,/\,min\,/\,m^{2=})}{Hb\ (gm\,/\,dL) \times 1.39 \times (Arterial\ O_2\ Sat\% - Venous\ O_2\ Sat\%)}$

Stroke Volume $\quad = \dfrac{CO}{Heart\ Rate}$

Systemic Vascular Resistance $= \dfrac{80 \times (MAP(mm\ Hg) - Mean\ RA\ pressure)}{CO\ (L\,/\,min)}$ $\quad (Normal\ 770 - 1500\ dyne - sec - cm^{-5})$

Pulmonary Vascular Resistance (Normal 20 - 120) $= \dfrac{80 \times (Mean\ PA\ pressure - Mean\ PCWP)}{CO}$

Poiseuille law of laminar flow: $\quad Velocity = \dfrac{Pp \cdot r^4}{8hl}$

Body Surface Area: $\quad BSA\ (m^2) = Height\ (cm)^{0.718} \times Weight\ (kg)^{0.427} \times 74.5$

$\quad \approx \sqrt{(Height\ (cm) \times Weight\ (kg) \div 3600)}$

Pulmonary Equations

Alveolar O_2 estimate: $PAO_2 = FiO_2 \times [pAtmospheric - pH_2O] - \dfrac{pCO_2}{Resp\ Quotient}$

$$= FiO_2 \times [760 - 47\ mm\ Hg] - \dfrac{pCO_2}{0.8}$$

Alveolar - arterial O_2 gradient $= PAO_2 - PaO_2 \approx 2.5 + 0.21 \times Age\ (yrs)$ upright
PaO_2 upright $\approx 104.2 - 0.27 \times Age\ (yrs)$

PaO_2 supine $\approx 103.5 - 0.42 \times Age\ (yrs)$

$PaCO_2$ $\qquad = K \times \dfrac{CO_2\ Production}{Alveolar\ Ventilation} = 0.863 \times \dfrac{VCO_2}{VA}$

Tidal Volume: $\qquad V_T = (V_{dead\ space} + V_{alveolar\ space}) = V_D + V_A$

Minute Ventilation: $\qquad VE = \dfrac{0.863 \times VCO_2\ (ml/min)}{PaCO_2 \times (1 - VD/V_T)}$ (Normal 4 - 6 L/min)

Bohr Dead Space: $\quad \dfrac{VD}{V_T} = \dfrac{PACO_2 - Pexpired\ CO_2}{PACO_2}$ (Normal 0.2 - 0.3)

Physiologic Dead Space: $\dfrac{VD}{V_T} = \dfrac{PACO_2 - Pexpired\ CO_2}{PaCO_2}$

Static Compliance $= \dfrac{V_T}{Pplateau - Pend\ expiration}$ (Normal > 60 mL/cm H_2O)

Dynamic Compliance $= \dfrac{V_T}{Ppeak - Pend\ expiration}$ (Normal > 60 mL/cm H_2O)

LaPlace law of surface tension: $\quad Pressure = \dfrac{2 \times Tension}{Radius}$

O_2 Dissolved in blood: $\qquad DO_2 = 0.0031 \times PaO_2\ (mm\ Hg)$

O_2 Content of blood: $\qquad CO_2 = DO_2 + 1.36 \times Hb\ (gm/dL) \times (O_2\ Sat\ \%)$
(Normal 17.5 - 23.5 mL/dL)

$R \rightarrow L$ Shunt: $\dfrac{Qs}{Qt} = \dfrac{CcO_2 - CaO_2}{CcO_2 - CvO_2} = \dfrac{(A - aDO_2) \times 0.0031}{(A - aDO_2) \times 0.0031 - CaO_2 - CvO_2}$

$R \rightarrow L$ Shunt on FiO_2 1.0: $\dfrac{Qs}{Qt} = \dfrac{(A - aDO_2)}{20}$ (Normal < 10%)

Medical "Statistics"

	Disease Present	Disease Absent
Test Positive	TP	FP
Test Negative	FN	TN

Prevalence (prior probability) = (TP+FN)/(ALL) = all patients with dz / all pts
Sensitivity = TP / (TP + FN) = True positive / all diseased
Specificity = TN / (FP + TN) = True negative / all healthy
False positive rate = 1 - Specificity
False negative rate = 1 - Sensitivity
Positive predictive value = TP / (TP + FP) = True-positive / all positives
Negative predictive value = TN / (FN + TN) = True-negative / all negatives
Accuracy = (TP + TN) / (ALL) = True results / all patients

Pediatric Vitals[3]

Age	Awake HR	Asleep HR	Respiratory Rate	Systolic BP	Diastolic BP
Birth (12h,<1kg)				39-59	16-36
Birth (12h, 3kg)				50-70	25-45
Neonate (96hr)	100-180	80-60		60-90	20-60
Infant 6mo	100-160	75-160	30-60	87-105	53-66
Toddler 2yr	80-110	60-90	24-40	95-108	53-66
Preschooler	70-110	60-90	22-34	96-110	55-69
School-age child 7yr	65-110	60-90	18-30	97-112	57-71
Adolescent 15 yr	60-90	50-90	12-16	112-128	66-80

---

[3] Cummins RO (ed.), Textbook of Advanced Cardiac Life Support, Dallas: American Heart Association, 1994, page 1:65.

Critical Care

ACLS V-Fib & Pulseless V-Tach[4]

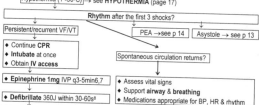

- ◆ Airway/Breathing/Circulation
- ◆ CPR until defibrillator available (Witnessed → Consider precordial **thump**[5])
- ◆ VF/VT present on monitor?

Defibrillate up to 3 times for persistent VF/VT (200J, 200-300J, 360J)

Hypothermia (T<30ºC) → see HYPOTHERMIA (page 17)

Rhythm after the first 3 shocks?

Persistent/recurrent VF/VT   PEA →see p 14   Asystole → see p 13

- ◆ Continue **CPR**
- ◆ **Intubate** at once
- ◆ Obtain **IV** access

Spontaneous circulation returns?

- ◆ **Epinephrine** 1mg IVP q3-5min,6,7

- ◆ Assess vital signs
- ◆ Support **airway** & breathing
- ◆ Medications appropriate for BP, HR & rhythm

- ◆ **Defibrillate** 360J within 30-60s[8]

Administer medications with probable benefit (Class IIa) in persistent/recurrent VF/VT:
- ◆ **Lidocaine** 1.5 mg/kg IVP. Repeat q 3-5 min to total 3mg/kg; then use
- ◆ **Bretylium** 5 mg/kg IVP. Repeat in 5 min at 10 mg/kg
- ◆ **Magnesium sulfate** 1-2g IVP:Torsades de pointes, suspected ↓ Mg, severe refractory VF
- ◆ **Procainamide** 30 mg/min in refractory VF (maximum total 17 mg/kg)
- ◆ **Amiodarone**[9] 150 mg IV over 10 min then 1 mg/min x 6 hr then 0.5 mg/min x 18 hr.
- ◆ **Sodium bicarbonate** 1mEq/kg IVP

    Class I: ◆ Known hyperkalemia

    Class IIa: ◆ Known prexisting bicarbonate-responsive acidosis
                 ◆ Tricyclic antidepressant overdose; ◆ To alkalinize urine in drug OD

    Class IIb: ◆ If intubated and continued long arrest interval;
                 ◆ Upon return of spontaneous circulation after long arrest interval

    Class III: ◆ Hypoxic lactic acidosis

- ◆ **Defibrillate** 360J, 30-60s after each dose of medication, as **drug-shock, drug-shock**

---

[4] "Guidelines for cardiopulmonary resuscitation and emergency care," JAMA, 1992;268:2171-2302, Copyright 1992, American Medical Association, with permission.   Class I: definitely helpful; Class IIa: acceptable, probably helpful; Class IIb: acceptable, possibly harmful; Class III: not indicated, may be harmful.
[5] **Precordial thump** is Class IIb in witnessed arrest, no pulse, and no defibrillator immediately available.
[6] If this epi dose fails, consider these Class IIb dosing regimens: ◆ Intermediate: **Epinephrine** 2-5 mg IVP q 3-5 min. ◆ Escalating: **Epi** 1mg - 3 mg - 5 mg IVP q 3 min ◆ High: **Epi** 0.1 mg/kg IVP q 3-5 min.
[7] **Sodium bicarbonate** 1mEq/kg IVP is Class I if patient has known preexisting hyperkalemia.
[8] Multiple sequenced shocks are Class I, especially when medications are delayed.
[9] Not included in 1992 ACLS recommendations; FDA approved 1996.

ACLS Tachycardia[10]

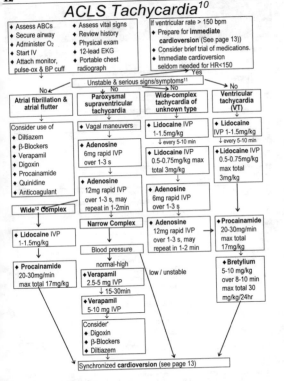

♦ Assess ABCs
♦ Secure airway
♦ Administer O₂
♦ Start IV
♦ Attach monitor, pulse-ox & BP cuff

♦ Assess vital signs
♦ Review history
♦ Physical exam
♦ 12-lead EKG
♦ Portable chest radiograph

If ventricular rate > 150 bpm
♦ Prepare for immediate cardioversion (See page 13))
♦ Consider brief trial of medications.
♦ Immediate cardioversion seldom needed for HR<150

Yes

Unstable & serious signs/symptoms[11]

No ──→ No ──→ No ──→ Yes

Atrial fibrillation & atrial flutter

Paroxysmal supraventricular tachycardia

Wide-complex tachycardia of unknown type

Ventricular tachycardia (VT)

Atrial fibrillation & atrial flutter

Consider use of
♦ Diltiazem
♦ β-Blockers
♦ Verapamil
♦ Digoxin
♦ Procainamide
♦ Quinidine
♦ Anticoagulant

Wide[12] Complex

♦ **Lidocaine** IVP 1-1.5mg/kg

♦ **Procainamide** 20-30mg/min max total 17mg/kg

Paroxysmal supraventricular tachycardia

♦ Vagal maneuvers

♦ **Adenosine** 6mg rapid IVP over 1-3 s

♦ **Adenosine** 12mg rapid IVP over 1-3 s, may repeat in 1-2min

Narrow Complex

Blood pressure

normal-high

♦ **Verapamil** 2.5-5 mg IVP
↓ 15-30min
♦ **Verapamil** 5-10 mg IVP

Consider*
♦ Digoxin
♦ β-Blockers
♦ Diltiazem

low / unstable

Wide-complex tachycardia of unknown type

♦ **Lidocaine** IVP 1-1.5mg/kg
↓ every 5-10 min
♦ **Lidocaine** IVP 0.5-0.75mg/kg max total 3mg/kg

♦ **Adenosine** 6mg rapid IVP over 1-3 s

♦ **Adenosine** 12mg rapid IVP over 1-3 s, may repeat in 1-2 min

---

Ventricular tachycardia (VT)

♦ **Lidocaine** IVP 1-1.5mg/kg
↓ every 5-10 min
♦ **Lidocaine** IVP 0.5-0.75mg/kg max total 3mg/kg

♦ **Procainamide** 20-30mg/min max total 17mg/kg

♦ **Bretylium** 5-10 mg/kg over 8-10 min max total 30 mg/kg/24hr

---

Synchronized **cardioversion** (see page 13)

---

[10] "Guidelines for cardiopulmonary resuscitation and emergency care", *JAMA*, 1992;268:2171-2302, Copyright 1992, American Medical Association, with permission.
[11] Unstable condition must be related to the tachycardia. Signs/symptoms may include chest pain, dyspnea, decreased consciousness, low BP, shock, pulmonary congestion, congestive heart failure, and acute MI.
[12] If wide complex rhythm is known with **certainty** to be PSVT and BP is acceptable, sequence can include verapamil. * Use extreme caution with β-blockers after verapamil or diltiazem.

ACLS Cardioversion for Tachycardia[13]

Tachycardia causing serious signs and symptoms

If ventricular rate is > 150 bpm, prepare for immediate cardioversion. May give brief trial of medications based on specific arrhythmias. Immediate cardioversion generally is **not** required for rates < 150 bpm.

| Check | ◆ Oxygen saturation | ◆ IV line |
| | ◆ Suction device | ◆ Intubation equipment |

Premedicate whenever possible[14]

Energy levels: Synchronized cardioversion:[15]

Polymorphic VT (irregular form & rate)	200J, 200-300J, 360J
VT (monomorphic), Atrial fibrillation	100J, 200J, 300J, 360J
PSVT, Atrial flutter	50J, 100J, 200J, 300J, 360J

ACLS Asystole[16]

◆ Continue CPR
◆ Intubate at once
◆ Obtain IV access
◆ Confirm asystole in more than one ECG lead

Consider possible causes.
◆ Hypoxia ◆ Hypokalemia
◆ Hyperkalemia
◆ Preexisting acidosis
◆ Drug overdose
◆ Hypothermia

Consider immediate **transcutaneous pacing (TCP)**[17]

◆ **Epinephrine** 1 mg IV push[18] q 3-5 min ◆ Consider bicarbonate[19]

◆ **Atropine** 1 mg IV q 3-5 min up to a total of 0.04 mg/kg[20]

◆ Consider **bicarbonate**[21]

Consider ◆ Termination of efforts[22]

---

[13] With the patient not in cardiac arrest. "Guidelines for cardiopulmonary resuscitation and emergency care," JAMA, 1992;268:2171-2302, Copyright 1992, American Medical Association, with permission.
[14] Effective regimens have included a sedative (eg, diazepam, midazolam, barbiturates, etomidate, ketamine, methohexital) with or without an analgesic (eg, fentanyl, morphine, meperidine). Many experts recommend anesthesiology assistance if service is readily available.
[15] Not possible need to resynchronize after each cardioversion. If delays in synchronization occur and clinical conditions are critical, go to immediate unsynchronized shocks.
[16] "Guidelines for cardiopulmonary resuscitation and emergency care," JAMA, 1992;268:2171-2302, Copyright 1992, American Medical Association, with permission. Class I: definitely helpful; Class IIa: acceptable, probably helpful; Class IIb: acceptable, possibly harmful; Class III: not indicated, may be harmful.
[17] TCP is a Class IIb intervention. Lack of success may be due to delays in pacing. To be effective, TCP must be performed early, simultaneously with drugs. Evidence does not support routine TCP for asystole.
[18] If this Epinephrine dose fails, consider several Class IIb dosing regimens: ◆ Intermediate: Epi 2-5 mg IVP q 3-5 min. ◆ Escalating: Epi 1mg - 3 mg - 5 mg IVP q 3 min ◆ High: Epi 0.1 mg/kg IVP q 3-5 min/
[19] Sodium bicarbonate 1mEq/kg IVP is Class I if patient has known preexisting hyperkalemia.
[20] Shorter dosing intervals are possibly helpful in cardiac arrest (Class IIb).
[21] Sodium bicarbonate 1mEq/kg IVP: Class IIa: ◆ Known preexisting bicarb-responsive acidosis ◆ Tricyclic antidepressant overdose; ◆ To alkalinize urine in drug OD   Class IIb: ◆ Intubated & long arrest interval; Class III: ◆ Hypoxic lactic acidosis
[22] Upon return of spontaneous circulation after long arrest interval. If asystole or other agonal rhythm persists after successful intubation and initial medications and no reversible causes are identified, consider MD termination of resuscitation. Consider the interval since arrest.

ACLS Pulseless Electrical Activity[23]

PEA (Electromechanical Dissociation) includes[24]

- Electromechanical dissocation (EMD)
- Pseudo-EMD
- Idioventricular rhythms
- Ventricular escape rhythms
- Bradyasystolic rhythms
- Postdefibrillation idioventricular rhythms

Management

- Continue CPR
- Intubate at once
- Obtain IV access
- Assess blood flow using handheld Doppler

Consider possible causes
- Hypovolemia → volume infusion
- Hypoxia → ventilation
- Cardiac tamponade →pericardiocentesis
- Tension pneumothorax → needle decompression
- Massive pulmonary thromboembolism → surgery, **thrombolytics**
- Drug overdoses such as tricyclics, digitalis, β-blockers, Ca-channel blockers
- Hyperkalemia[25]
- Acidosis[26]
- Hypothermia → (See page 16)
- Massive acute myocardial infarction

- **Epinephrine**[27] 1 mg IV push, repeat every 3-5 min   • Consider **bicarbonate**[28]

- If absolute (<60 bpm) or relative bradycardia, give **atropine** 1 mg IV
- Repeat every 3-5 min up to a total of 004 mg/kg[a]

ACLS Causes of Hypotension[29]

Rate problems

- <u>Too slow (see **bradycardia** on page 16)</u>: • Sinus bradycardia •Type II and II second-degree heart block • Third-degree heart block • Pacemaker failures
- <u>Too fast (see **tachycardia** on page 12)</u>: • Sinus tachycardia • Atrial flutter • Atrial fibrillation • Multifocal atrial tachycardia • Paroxysmal SVT • VT

Pump problems

- <u>Primary:</u> • Myocardial infarction • Cardiomyopathy • Myocarditis
- Acute valvular insufficiency: • Ruptured chordae tendinae • Acute papillary muscle dysfunction • Acute aortic insufficiency • Ruptured interventricular septum
- <u>Secondary:</u> • Negative inotropes (eg β-blockers, Ca-blockers) • Cardiac tamponade
- Pulmonary thromboembolism • Atrial myxoma • Superior vena cava syndrome

Volume problems

- <u>Absolute:</u> • Hemorrhage • Gastrointestinal loss • Renal loss • Insensible loss
- Adrenal insufficiency (aldosterone)
- <u>Relative (vasodilation or redistribution):</u> • Spinal or Central nervous system injury •Third-space loss • Tension pneumothorax • Adrenal insufficiency (cortisol) • Sepsis
- Drugs that alter vascular tone

---

[23] "Guidelines for cardiopulmonary resuscitation and emergency care," JAMA, 1992;268:2171-2302, Copyright 1992, American Medical Association, with permission.

[24] Class I: definitely helpful; Class IIa: acceptable, probably helpful; Class IIb: acceptable, possibly harmful; Class III: not indicated, may be harmful.

[25] **Sodium bicarbonate** 1mEq/kg IVP is Class I if patient has known preexisting hyperkalemia.

[26] **Sodium bicarbonate** IVP: Class IIa: • Known prexisting bicarb-responsive acidosis • Tricyclic antidepressant overdose; • To alkalinize urine in drug OD Class IIb: • Intubated & long arrest interval; • Upon return of spontaneous circulation after long arrest interval. Class III: • Hypoxic lactic acidosis

[27] If this epi dose fails, consider several Class IIb dosing regimens: • Intermediate: **Epinephrine** 2-5 mg IVP q 3-5 min. • Escalating: **Epi** 1mg - 3 mg - 5 mg IVP q 3 min • High: **Epi** 0.1 mg/kg IVP q 3-5 min.

[28] Shorter atropine dosing intervals are possibly helpful in cardiac arrest (Class IIb)

[29] "Guidelines for cardiopulmonary resuscitation and emergency care," JAMA, 1992;268:2171-2302, Copyright 1992, American Medical Association, with permission.

ACLS Hypotension & Pulmonary Edema[30]

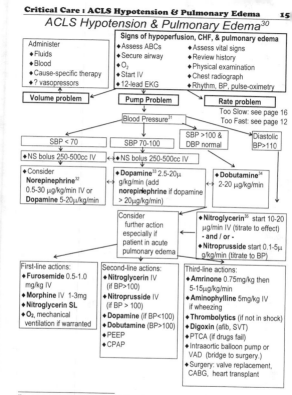

Administer
◆ Fluids
◆ Blood
◆ Cause-specific therapy
◆ ? vasopressors

Signs of hypoperfusion, CHF, & pulmonary edema
◆ Assess ABCs   ◆ Assess vital signs
◆ Secure airway   ◆ Review history
◆ O_2 ◆ Physical examination
◆ Start IV   ◆ Chest radiograph
◆ 12-lead EKG   ◆ Rhythm, BP, pulse-oximetry

Volume problem ← **Pump Problem** → **Rate problem**

Rate problem:
Too Slow: see page 16
Too Fast: see page 12

Blood Pressure[31]

SBP < 70	SBP 70-100	SBP >100 & DBP normal	Diastolic BP>110
◆ NS bolus 250-500cc IV	◆ NS bolus 250-500cc IV		
◆ Consider **Norepinephrine**[32] 0.5-30 µg/kg/min IV or **Dopamine** 5-20µg/kg/min	◆ **Dopamine**[33] 2.5-20µ g/kg/min (add norepinephrine if dopamine > 20µg/kg/min)	◆ **Dobutamine**[34] 2-20 µg/kg/min	

Consider further action especially if patient in acute pulmonary edema

◆ **Nitroglycerin**[35] start 10-20 µg/min IV (titrate to effect)
- and / or -
◆ **Nitroprusside** start 0.1-5µ g/kg/min (titrate to BP)

First-line actions:	Second-line actions:	Third-line actions:
◆ **Furosemide** 0.5-1.0 mg/kg IV	◆ **Nitroglycerin** IV (if BP>100)	◆ **Amrinone** 0.75mg/kg then 5-15µg/kg/min
◆ **Morphine** IV 1-3mg	◆ **Nitroprusside** IV (if BP > 100)	◆ **Aminophylline** 5mg/kg IV if wheezing
◆ **Nitroglycerin** SL	◆ **Dopamine** (if BP<100)	◆ **Thrombolytics** (if not in shock)
◆ O_2, mechanical ventilation if warranted	◆ **Dobutamine** (BP>100)	◆ **Digoxin** (afib, SVT)
	◆ PEEP	◆ PTCA (if drugs fail)
	◆ CPAP	◆ Intraaortic balloon pump or VAD (bridge to surgery.)
		◆ Surgery: valve replacement, CABG, heart transplant

---

[30] "Guidelines for cardiopulmonary resuscitation and emergency care," <u>JAMA</u>, 1992;268:2171-2302, Copyright 1992, American Medical Association, with permission.
[31] Further management should be based on invasive hemodynamic monitoring if possible.
[32] **Norepinephrine** (Levophed)
[33] Move to **dopamine** and stop **norepinephrine** when BP improves.
[34] Add **dopamine** when BP improves. Avoid **dobutamine** when SBP<100mm Hg.
[35] Use **nitroglycerin** if ischemia persists and BP remains elevated.

ACLS Bradycardia[36]

◆ Assess ABCs	◆ Assess vital signs
◆ Secure airway	◆ Review history
◆ Administer oxygen	◆ Perform physical examination
◆ Start IV	◆ Order 12-lead ECG
◆ Attach monitor, pulse-ox, and automatic sphygmomanometer	◆ Order portable chest roentgenogram

Too slow (<60 bpm)

Bradycardia, either absolute (<60bpm) or relative

Serious signs or symptoms related to slow rate:[37]
 Symptoms: chest pain, dyspnea, ↓ level of consciousness
 Signs: Low BP, shock, pulmonary congestion, CHF, acute MI

No ←——————————→ Yes

Type II second-degree AV block?
 - or -
Third-degree AV heart block?

No   Yes

◆ Observe

Intervention sequence:
◆ **Atropine** 0.5-1.0 mg q 3-5 min (I&IIa) [38,39]
◆ TCP if available (I)
◆ **Dopamine** 5-20 µg/kg/min (IIb)
◆ **Epinephrine** 2-10 µg/kg/min (IIb)
◆ **Isoproterenol** [40]

◆ Prepare for transvenous pacemaker
◆ Use **transcutaneous pacing** as a bridge device [41]

ACLS Emergency Cardiac Pacing[42]

Indications for Emergency Pacing

◆ Hemodynamically compromising bradycardias: (BP < 80mm systolic, change in mental status, myocardial ischemia, pulmonary edema)
 Includes complete heart block, symptomatic second-degree heart block, symptomatic sick sinus syndrome, drug-induced bradycardias (ie, digoxin, β-blockers, calcium channel blockers, or procainamide), permanent pacemaker failure, idioventricular bradycardias, symptomatic atrial fibrillation with slow ventricular response, refractory bradycardia during resuscitation of hypovolemic shock, and bradyarrhythmias with malignant ventricular escape mechanisms

◆ Bradycardia with malignant escape rhythms (unresponsive to drug therapy)

◆ Overdrive pacing of refractory tachycardia: Supraventricular or ventricular (currently indicated only in special situations refractory to drugs or cardioversion)

◆ Bradyasystolic cardiac arrest: Pacing not routinely recommended. If used at all, pacing should be used as early as possible after onset of arrest

---

[36] With patient not in cardiac arrest. "Guidelines for cardiopulmonary resuscitation and emergency care," JAMA, 1992;268:2171-2302, Copyright 1992, American Medical Association, with permission.
[37] Do not delay TCP while awaiting IV access or for **atropine** to take effect if the patient is symptomatic.
[38] **Atropine** should be given in repeat doses in 3-5 min up to total of 0.04 mg/kg. Consider shorter dosing intervals in severe clinical conditions. It has been suggested that atropine should be used with caution in atrioventricular (AV) block at the His-Purkinje level (Type II AV block and new third-degree block with wide QRS complexes) (Class IIb).
[40] Denervated, transplanted hearts will not respond to **atropine**. Use pacing, **catecholamines**, or both.
[40] **Isoproterenol** should be used, if at all, with extreme caution. At low doses it is Class IIb (possibly helpful); at higher doses it is Class III (harmful).
[41] Verify patient tolerance of TCP as well as mechanical capture. Use analgesia and sedation as needed.
[42] "Guidelines for cardiopulmonary resuscitation and emergency care," JAMA, 1992;268:2171-2302, Copyright 1992, American Medical Association, with permission.

Technique
See "Cardiology: Emergency cardiac pacing," page 36.

Standby pacing
- Stable bradycardias (BP > 80mm Hg, no evidence of hemodynamic compromise, or hemodynamic compromise responsive to initial drug therapy)
- Prophylactic pacing in acute myocardial infarction: • Symptomatic sinus node dysfunction • Mobitz II second-degree heart block • Third-degree heart block • Newly acquired left bundle-branch block, right bundle-branch block, alternating bundle-branch block, or bifascicular block

ACLS Hypothermia[43]

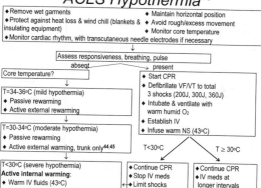

- Remove wet garments
- Protect against heat loss & wind chill (blankets & insulating equipment)
- Monitor cardiac rhythm, with transcutaneous needle electrodes if necessary
- Maintain horizontal position
- Avoid rough/excess movement
- Monitor core temperature

Assess responsiveness, breathing, pulse

absent → **present**

absent:

Core temperature?

T=34-36°C (mild hypothermia)
- Passive rewarming
- Active external rewarming

T=30-34°C (moderate hypothermia)
- Passive rewarming
- Active external warming, trunk only[44,45]

T<30°C (severe hypothermia)
Active internal warming:
- Warm IV fluids (43°C)
- Warm, humid O$_2$ (42-46°C)
- Peritoneal lavage (KCl-free fluid)
- Extracorporeal warming
- Esophageal rewarming tubes[46]

Continue internal rewarming until:
- Core temperature ≥ 35°C
- Return of spontaneous circulation
- Resuscitative efforts cease

present:
- Start CPR
- Defibrillate VF/VT to total 3 shocks (200J, 300J, 360J)
- Intubate & ventilate with warm humid O$_2$
- Establish IV
- Infuse warm NS (43°C)

T<30°C
- Continue CPR
- Stop IV meds
- Limit shocks for VF/VT to 3
- Transport to hospital

T ≥ 30°C
- Continue CPR
- IV meds at longer intervals
- Repeat defib for VF/VT as Temp rises

---

[43] "Guidelines for cardiopulmonary resuscitation and emergency care," JAMA, 1992;268:2171-2302, Copyright 1992, American Medical Association, with permission.
[44] Many experts think these interventions should be done only in-hospital, though practices vary
[45] Methods include electric or charcoal warming devices, hot water bottles, heating pads, radiant heat sources, and warming beds
[46] Esophageal rewarming tubes are widely used internationally and should become available in the US

Swan-Ganz PA Catheters[47]

Utility • Distinguish between cardiogenic (CHF, tamponade) and noncardiogenic (cor pulmonale, ARDS) pulmonary edema. • Guide therapy to improve LV filling or decrease pulmonary edema (eg, complicated myocardial infarction, shock, ARDS, uncertain intravascular volume in critically ill patient). • Measure cardiac output, O_2 saturation; infer SVR & PVR.

Verify PCWP position:
- Characteristic waveforms with balloon in/deflation
- PCWP < PADP; mean PCWP < mean PAP
- Continuous flush shows no tip obstruction
- Blood from catheter tip is 100% saturated in absence of pulmonary disease or shunt (Sample "wedge sat" with balloon inflated after discarding 5cc)

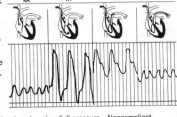

RA   RV   PA   PCWP

High LVEDP may represent:
- High extracardiac (thoracic, pleural, pericardial) pressure • Noncompliant ventricle (diastolic dysfunction) • ↑ distention of normal-compliant ventricle (CHF)

PCWP misrepresents LVEDP when
- Intrapericardial/intrathoracic pressure is high (eg obstructive lung disease). Note LVEDP = intracardiac - intrapericardial pressure, while PCWP = intracardiac - atmospheric pressure.
- Catheter in non "Zone III" position: "overwedged" waveform, PCWP>PAD Balloon floats anteriorly in supine patients; Hypovolemia changes Zone III to Zone I/II   PEEP changes Zone III to Zone I-II
- Hypovolemia: PCWP especially sensitive to fluctuations in PA vascular tone
- "Catheter whip" esp in hyperdynamic states • Valvular disease (MR, MS, AI with early mitral closure) • Tachycardia shortens diastolic filling • Obstruction to catheter tip (mediastinal fibrosis, myxoma, tumors)

PA diastolic may exceed PCWP & LVEDP:
- Elevated PVR: Thrombotic occlusion (PE); Hypoxic vasoconstriction; Parenchymal disorders: COPD, pulmonary hypertension • Tachycardia

"Physiologic" LVEDP is rate-dependent, since CO=HR×SV
Bradycardias ↑ LVEDP; Tachycardias ↓ LVEDP

High LVEDP does not predict pulmonary edema since Chronic congestion increases lymphatic drainage and decreases vascular permeability.   Endothelial injury causes edema at normal LVEDP.

Special cases
- PEEP: Typically correct PCWP by subtracting ½ of PEEP: PCWP proportionate to LVEDP, for PEEP < 10;   RAP proportionate to LVEDP for PEEP > 10

---

[47] O'Quin R & Marini J "PAOP: clinical physiology, measurement, and interpretation," <u>Am Rev Respir Dis</u> 128:319, 1983; Sharkey S, "Beyond the wedge: clinical physiology and the Swan-Ganz catheter," <u>Am J Med</u> 83:111, 1987; Wiedemann HP, Matthay M, Matthay R, "Cardiovascular-pulmonary monitoring in the ICU," <u>Chest</u> 85: 537-49, 656-68, 1984; Connors A et al, "Hemodynamic status in critically ill patients with and without acute heart disease," <u>Chest</u> 98:1200, 1990. Figures copyright 1987 Lawrence Martin MD, with permission.

- **Mitral regurgitation:**
  Measure with simultaneous QRS. <u>Balloon deflation</u>: bifid PA systolic & regurgitant V wave.
  <u>Balloon inflation</u>: Giant V-wave, moves "later" relative to QRS complex; A-wave obliterated.
  Oxygenated blood may regurgitate into PA.

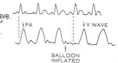

Central vein anomalies[48]

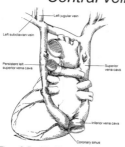

Figure 2. Persistent L superior vena cava

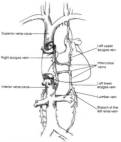

Figure 1. 'Typical' azygos anatomy

Here the L subclavian and jugular veins drain into the left SVC rather than the L brachiocephalic vein. The L SVC drains into the coronary sinus via the oblique vein. Seen in 0.3% normals; 4.5% of pts with congenital heart disease.

Azygos variations are common. The R azygos can arise from a branch of the right renal vein, one of the R lumbar veins, or from the IVC. The R azygos joins the SVC via either the aortic hiatus or the R diaphragmatic crus.

Using Mechanical Ventilators[49]

Patients with normal lung mechanics & gas exchange
- ◆ Indications: • Loss of central drive to breath (*eg* drug overdose, brainstem injury) • Neuromuscular weakness • Adjunctive therapy for shock
  • Hyperventilation following brain injury
- ◆ Settings: FiO_2 0.21-0.40; Tidal volume 8-12 mL/kg; Rate 8-12/min (18-24/min for therapeutic hyperventilation, high enough to cease respiratory efforts in shock); Peak flow 40 L/min adjusted to comfort; SIMV or AC with minimal (-2cm H_2O) sensitivity, PS mode in neuromuscular dz

---

[48] PG Polos, SA Sahn, "Tips for monitoring the position of a central venous catheter," <u>J Crit Illness</u>, 1993;8(6):660.

[49] Adapted with permission from JB Hall and LDH Wood "Management of the patient on a ventilator," pp 1617-1633 in Hall, Schmidt, & Wood (eds.), <u>Principles of Critical Care</u>, NY: McGraw-Hill, 1992, Copyright 1992 McGraw-Hill.

◆ Things to consider
- Target P_aCO_2 of 25 torr if goal is reduction of intracranial pressure.
- In shock, Use higher minute ventilation or sedation/muscle relaxation.
- Prevent atelectasis: 3-pt turning; physiotherapy; sighs; low-level PEEP
- Peak airway pressure should be < 30 cmH_2O

Severe airflow obstruction
◆ Indications: Status asthmaticus; Thermal injury of the upper airway; Central airway obstruction by mass; Tracheal stenosis
◆ Settings: F_iO_2 .30-.50 (higher requirements suggest alveolar disease); Tidal volume 5-7 mL/kg; Rate 15-18/min; Peak flow 60 L/min (in effort to lengthen expiratory time); Controlled mode (or AC/SIMV with high mandatory rate)
◆ Things to consider:
- Diminished venous return common on initiation of mechanical ventilation; **hypotension** responds to volume or to temporarily disconnecting ventilator.
- Early sedation and muscle relaxation will ↓ discomfort, ↓ airway pressure, and ↓ O_2 consumption.
- Maintain peak airway pressure < 55 cmH_2O to minimize **barotrauma**
- **Intrinsic PEEP** ("auto-PEEP") reflects elevated alveolar pressure at end-expiration in severe airway obstruction. It is measured at the airway opening during an expiratory hold maneuver while occluding the expiratory & inspiratory limbs of the ventilator. Intrinsic PEEP is exacerbated by shortened expiratory time. $PEEP_i$ effectively raises pressure needed to trigger ventilator, requires much work, and potentiates muscle fatigue. Keep intrinsic PEEP < 15 cm H_2O
- Intentional hypoventilation (permissive hypercapnea) may be preferable to gas trapping intrinsic PEEP and high airway pressures. Note some investigators even infuse bicarbonate to minimize acidemia.
- PEEP and sighs are undesirable since pressures are already excessive

Acute-on-chronic respiratory failure
◆ Indications: Progessive respiratory muscle fatigue
◆ Settings: F_iO_2 0.25-0.40 (higher requirements suggest alveolar process); Tidal volume 6-8 mL/kg; Rate 15-18/min; Mode SIMV or AC; Adjust inspiratory flow rates to resolve patient dyspnea
◆ Things to consider:
- Complete rest for 36-72 h
- Hypotension common after instituting mechanical ventilation (see above)
- Post-intubation alkalemia is common in face of chronic resp acidosis; ventilation to P_aCO_2 lower than baseline may interfere with weaning
- Continued effort from triggering the ventilator with in the presence of intrinsic-PEEP may prevent resolution of fatigue (see above)
- PEEP or CPAP may be beneficial when pt begins respiratory muscle exercise

Acute hypoxemic respiratory failure
◆ Indications: Inadequate arterial Hb saturation via O_2 and positive pressure delivered by mask, and/or tachypnea and dyspnea predicting imminent respiratory muscle fatigue.
◆ Causes of hypoxemia • V/Q mismatch, • Shunt • Inadequate F_iO_2
- Hypoventilation • Diffusion impairment
◆ Settings: F_iO_2 initially 1.0; Tidal volume 6-7 mL/kg; Rate 24-28/min; SIMV or AC with minimal (-2 cmH_2O) sensitivity; PEEP titrated as below.
◆ Things to consider:
- **PEEP** redistributes fluid from alveolar to interstitial compartments, and recruits collapsed/flooded alveoli.
- Determining minimum/"optimal" PEEP:
- Add PEEP in 5 cmH_2O increments

- Measure **compliance** [C = Tidal Volume / (Static pressure - PEEP)] 30-60s after each change; also measure BP and S_aO_2
- If compliance increases, then add additional PEEP and repeat; If compliance "plateaus," additional PEEP has no benefit
- PEEP may interfere with RA/LA filling, causing hypotension/tachycardia
- In inhomogenous lung disease (eg lobar pneumonia), PEEP may not improve and may increase intrapulmonary shunt
- Interrupting PEEP circuit even transiently can cause deterioration
- $F_iO_2 > 0.6$ may cause diffuse alveolar damage; Use minimum PEEP to achieve $S_aO_2 > 90\%$ of adequate Hb using a nontoxic $F_iO_2 < 0.6$.
- Attain <u>minimum PCWP</u> that achieves an adequate cardiac output
- <u>Barotrauma</u> may potentiate underlying alveolar damage
- Recent interest in inverse-ratio and high-frequency ventilation

Restrictive lung disease

◆ Indications: • Acute insult (eg pneumonia) or complicating restrictive lung (eg pulmonary fibrosis) or chest wall (eg kyphoscoliosis) disease. • Proliferative-phase ARDS. • Rarely, massive and tense fluid collection in the abdomen, or s/p abdominal surgery.

◆ Settings: F_iO_2 .30-.50; tidal volume 6-7 mL/kg; rate18-24/min; mode SIMV or AC

◆ Things to consider:
- Relieve restriction if possible (eg paracentesis, escharotomy)
- Note benefit of upright posture in intraabdominal processes
- These patients prone to increased physiologic dead space from high minute ventilation and PEEP, especially with concurrent hypovolemia (from expansion of West "Zone I"), and to reduced venous return impairing cardiac output.

Indications for sedation and muscle relaxation

- Hypoperfusion with lactic acidosis
- Status asthmaticus or other airway disease with high airway pressure and intrinsic PEEP
- Acute hypoxemic respiratory failure and instability or toxic F_iO_2 despite PEEP
- Control of central neurogenic hyperventilation
- Acute hypoxemic respiratory failure with high intrinsic PEEP and struggling
- High-risk of barotrauma, including bronchopleural fistula in pts with chest tubes

Noninvasive (mask) ventilation[50] can preempt endotracheal intubation in alert patients with hypoxemic (ie congestive heart failure[51]) and hypercarbic respiratory failure (ie COPD decompensation), but requires skilled respiratory therapists and cooperative patients.

Ventilator emergencies

High pressure
- **Disconnect from ventilator and bag @ FiO2 100%!**
- Check external obstruction (biting or kinking endotracheal tube)
- Suction endotracheal tube and airway to remove mucus plugs and clots
- Examine for
- Biting endotracheal tube: introduce bite block, consider sedation or paralysis
- Tracheal obstruction: no air entry to lungs → urgent bronchoscopy

[50] Brochard L, et al, "Noninvasive ventilation for acute exacerbations of chronic obstructive pulmonary disease," N Engl J Med, 1995;333(13):817-22. Bott J, et al, "Randomised controlled trial of nasal ventilation in acute ventilatory failure due to chronic obstructive airways disease," Lancet, 1993;341(8860):1555-7. Kramer N, et al, "Randomized, prospective trial of noninvasive positive pressure ventilation in acute respiratory failure," Am J Respir Crit Care Med, 1995;151(6):1799-806. Meyer TJ, Hill NS, "Noninvasive positive pressure ventilation to treat respiratory failure," Ann Intern Med, 1994;120(9):760-70.
[51] Bersten AD, et al, "Treatment of severe cardiogenic pulmonary edema with continuous positive airway pressure delivered by face mask," N Engl J Med, 1991;325(26):1825-30.

- Bronchial obstruction: no expansion of affected lung → urgent bronchoscopy
- Wheezing suggesting small airways obstruction; note severe bronchospasm limits wheezing because of limited air movement → bronchodilators
- Pneumothorax: no chest excursion, expansion, hyperresonance, hypotension → needle & chest tube
- Endotracheal tube in R mainstem bronchus: exam similar to PTX

Low-pressure
- **Disconnect from ventilator and bag @ FiO2 100%!**
- Endotracheal tube slipped out of trachea -> reintubate
- Cuff leak -> instill more air into cuff; reintubate
- Tracheoesophageal fistula -> attempt to reposition tube
- Leak within mechanical ventilator

Weaning from Mechanical Ventilation

Predictors of successful weaning[52]

Test	Ventilator < 8 d[a]		Ventilator ≥ 8 days	
	Sensit'y	Specif'y	Sensit'y	Specif'y
Minute ventilation ≤ 15 L/min	.79	.75	.75	.08
Resp rate / Tidal volume ≤ 105/min-L	1.0	.63	.88	.67
Dynamic compliance ≥ 22 mL/cm H_2O	.75	.69	.63	.25
Static compliance ≥ 33 ml/cm H_2O	.82	.56	.50	.08
Tidal volume ≥ 325 mL	1.0	.50	.88	.58
Tidal volume ≥ 4 mL/kg	.96	.38	.88	.42
P_aO_2 / P_AO_2 ≥ 0.35	.79	.38	.88	.17
Resp rate ≤ 38/min	.89	.31	1.0	.42
Maximum insp pressure ≤ -15 cm H_2O	1.0	.00	1.0	.25

a: Duration of mechanical ventilation < 8 days.

"Traditional" predictors of successful weaning
- Negative inspiratory force (NIF) > 20 cm H_2O • Vital capacity > 10-15 ml / kg ideal body weight • Minute ventilation < 10 liters/min; • Maximum voluntary ventilation > 2×minute ventilation • Respiratory rate < 30 • P_aO_2 > 60 mm Hg with F_iO_2 < 0.40

Optimize before weaning:
- Sit patient upright; Suction pharynx thoroughly • Withdraw sedative drugs and ensure adequate rest • Psychological preparation of pt • Adequate nutrition • Minimize pulmonary edema with maximum diuresis • Reverse bronchospasm • Normalize electrolytes affecting muscle function eg, P, Mg, Ca, K • Optimize blood O_2-carrying capacity (eg transfuse to Hct>25-30%) • Suppress fever with antipyretics • Effectively treat systemic illnesses, (eg infections); Institute effective antianginal therapy • Consider "pressure support" ventilatory modes to overcome resistance of narrow endotracheal tubes • Consider possible drug-induced neuromuscular blockade, (eg aminoglycosides, residual pancuronium)

Weaning Modes: Controversial[53]
- Intermittent mandatory ventilation; • Pressure Support Ventilation; • Trials of spontaneous breathing through endotracheal tube

[52] KL Yang and MJ Tobin, "A prospective study of indexes predicting the outcome of trials of weaning from mechanical ventilation," N Engl J Med, 1991;324(21):1445-50.
[53] Esteban A, et al, "A comparison of four methods of weaning patients from mechanical ventilation. Spanish Lung Failure Collaborative Group," N Engl J Med 1995;332(6):345-50.

Hypercapnea

Alveolar gas equation
Explains differential diagnosis of hypercapnea. P_aCO_2 is increased by increased CO_2 production and by reduced alveolar ventilation:

$$V_A = V_E - V_D \qquad pCO_2 \approx \frac{V_{CO_2}}{V_A} \qquad \frac{V_D}{V_T} = \frac{P_aCO_2 - P_ECO_2}{P_aCO_2}$$

Where V_{CO_2} is CO_2 production; V_A is alveolar ventilation; V_E is minute ventilation; V_D is dead-space ventilation; V_T is tidal volume; P_ECO_2 is expired partial-pressure of CO_2.

Decreased minute ventilation
Central Hypoventilation
• Sleep apnea syndromes • Drug-induced respiratory depression (eg barbiturates, opiates) • Hypothyroidism • Brainstem disease

Neuromuscular & musculoskeletal weakness
• Respiratory muscle fatigue (eg acute-on-chronic resp failure, shock) • Drug-induced (eg pancuronium, aminoglycoside) • Chest wall disease (eg kyphoscoliosis, thoracoplasty, flail-chest, obesity) • Myasthenia gravis; Motor-neuron disease (ALS); muscular dystrophy; Post-polio syndrome; High cervical trauma

Increased dead-space ventilation
Obliteration of functional alveoli: • parenchymal disease, fibrosis, cyst formation
Interruption of alveolar vascular supply: • Pulmonary thromboembolism • Volume depletion (converts West Zone II-III lung to Zone I) • Positive-pressure ventilation & PEEP (- converts West Zone II-III lung to Zone I; - Diverts perfusion from healthy, compliant alveoli to diseases alveoli)

Excessive CO_2 production: eg, metabolic alkalosis

Oxygen. Induces hypercapnea in ventilatory failure:
• Reduces hypoxic ventilatory drive in pts with chronically-blunted hypercapneic ventilatory drive. **Probably not clinically relevant** in acute respiratory failure.
• Increased dead-space ventilation from O_2-mediated bronchodilation.
• Use oxygen judiciously in patients with hypercapnea, but remember that **hypoxemia is more dangerous than hypercapnea** in alert patients!

Right to Left Pulmonary Shunt[54]

Causes of shunt:
• Normal shunting via bronchial, mediastinal, Thebesian veins • Alveolar collapse (Atelectasis, consolidation) • Impaired gas diffusion • Severe ventilation-diffusion mismatch • Anatomic shunts eg pulmonary AV fistulae; intracardiac shunts eg VSD, PDA, ASD

Derivation
Cardiac output (Q_t) = Shunted blood flow (Q_s) - Oxygenated blood (Q_t-Q_s)
Arterial oxygen flux = Shunted oxygen flux + Nonshunted oxygen flux

$$Q_t \times C_aO_2 = Q_s \times C_vO_2 + [(Q_t-Q_s) \times C_cO_2]$$

Recall the formula for oxygen content:

$$C_xO_2 = [1.39 \times Hb\ (g/dL) \times (O_2\ sat\ \%)] + [.0031 \times P_aO_2]$$

Where C_cO_2 = Pulmonary capillary oxygen; C_aO_2 = Arterial O_2 content;
C_vO_2 = Mixed venous blood oxygen content (from PA catheter)

[54] L Martin, Pulmonary physiology in clinical practice, pp223-5, St. Louis: CV Mosby, 1987, with permission; Johnson JL, CWRU presentation.

$A\text{-}aDO_2$ = Alveolar - arterial oxygen difference

Rearranging gives the shunt fraction:

$$\frac{Q_s}{Q_t} = \frac{C_{cO_2} - C_{aO_2}}{C_{cO_2} - C_{vO_2}} \quad or \quad \frac{Q_s}{Q_t} = \frac{(A - aDO_2) \times 0.0031}{(A - aDO_2) \times 0.0031 - C_{aO_2} - C_{vO_2}}$$

Note F_iO_2 should > 0.6 to overcome areas of physiologic low V/Q. When F_iO_2=100%, C_cO_2 is assumed to be 100% saturated. With normal cardiac output, this reduces to:

$$\frac{Q_s}{Q_t} = \frac{(A - aDO_2) \times 0.0031}{C_aO_2 - C_vO_2} = \frac{A - a \text{ gradient (mmHg)}}{20}$$

Interpretation

<10%	Normal
10-20%	Moderate abnormality, usually can oxygenate spontaneously
20-30%	Severe shunt often requires high supplemental F_iO_2 or PEEP, may be life-threatening in patients with limited CNS or cardiopulmonary reserve
>30%	Big trouble

Poisoning: General Management[55]

Initial management
- Supportive, especially <u>Airway</u>: ? supplemental O_2, ? respiratory muscle strength
- Consider <u>Naloxone</u> 2mg (Respiratory depression, suspected of opiate ingestion)
- <u>Thiamine</u> 100mg (Chronic alcoholics)
- Consider <u>Dextrose 50%</u> (Suspected hypoglycemia)
- Consider <u>Flumazenil</u> 2.5mg IV then 0.1 mg/min total 5mg (Contraindicated in undefined overdose, TCA coingestion, seizure d/o, chronic benzodiazepine use)

Laboratory analysis
- Chemistry, anion gap, ABG, osmolality, ? lactate, ? toxicology screen including salicylate, acetaminophen, TCA, ethanol.
- (Measured-predicted) osmolal gap suggests alcohols (eg ethanol, methanol), ketones (eg acetone), sugars (eg mannitol).
- Lactic acidosis suggests seizure, hypoperfusion, cyanide, CO, etc.
- Pulse-oximetry does **NOT** reveal methemoglobinemia or CO poisoning; use (blood) co-oximetry instead!

Decontamination
- Intubate trachea to protect airway if consciousness is depressed
- Consider large-bore orogastric H_2O/NS lavage (until effluent clear) **unless** (1) corrosive or hydrocarbon ingestion; (2) sharp object; (3) coagulopathy. Many experts skip lavage and proceed directly to charcoal decontamination (below).
- Activated charcoal 0.5-1mg/kg q 4h. Use sorbitol 0.5-1mg/kg with first dose. Especially effective for large MW compounds. Avoid if GI dysmotility.
- Bowel irrigation (eg Golytely™) 1.5-2L/h until clear, if no GI dysmotility.
- Skin decontamination if warranted (eg radiation, insecticides)

Enhanced elimination
- **Diuresis**   • Saline: (eg lithium)
  - Alkaline (ie $NaHCO_3$ to urine pH 7.5-8): eg salicylate, barbiturates, rhabdo
- **Hemodialysis or hemoperfusion**
  - Indicated when supportive care is inadequate & drug can be cleared

[55] KR Olson, *et al*, "Physical assessment and differential diagnosis of the poisoned patient," <u>Med Toxicol</u>, 2:52, 1987; SM Pond, "Diuresis, dialysis and hemoperfusion," <u>Emerg Med Clin North Am</u>, 2:29, 1984. U Taitelman & MJ Ellenhorn, "General management of poisoning," in JB Hall *et al* (eds) "Principles of Critical Care," NY:McGraw-Hill, 1992.

- **Hemodialysis** removes alcohols, salicylates, lithium
- **Hemoperfusion** removes theophylline, phenobarbital

Specific Antidotes

Antidote	Indication	Antidote	Indication
Physostigmine	Anticholinergic syndrome	Methylene blue	Methemoglobin
Pralidoxime	Organophosphate	Deferoxamine	Iron
Flumazenil	Benzodiazepines	Digoxin Fab	Digitalis
Glucagon	β-blocker, Ca-blocker	N-acetylcysteine	Acetaminophen
Diphenhydramine	Dystonic reaction	Naloxone	Opiates
Ethanol 10%	Methanol, ethylene glycol	Pyridoxine	Isoniazid
Dantrolene	Malignant hyperthermia, neuroleptic malignant syndr.	Vitamin K	Warfarin
Leucovorin	Methanol, antifolates (eg methotrexate, trimethoprim)	Thiosulfate; Nitrite; Hydroxy-cobalamin	Cyanide

Common Toxic Syndromes[56]

Anticholinergic syndromes
- Common Signs: Delirium with mumbling speech, tachycardia, dry flushed skin, dilated pupils, myoclonus, slightly elevated temperature, urinary retention, and decreased bowel sounds. Seizures & dysrhythmias may occur in severe cases.
- Common causes: Antihistamines, antiparkinsonian medication, atropine, scopolamine, amantadine, antipsychotic agents, antidepressant agents, antispasmodic agents, mydriatic agents, skeletal muscle relaxants, many plants (most notably jimson weed and *Amanita muscaria*).

Sympathomimetic syndromes
- Common signs: Delusions, paranoia, tachycardia (or bradycardia if the drug is a pure α-adrenergic agonist), hypertension, hyperpyrexia, diaphoresis, piloerection, mydriasis, and hyperreflexia. Seizures, hypotension, and dysrhythmias may occur in severe cases.
- Common causes: Cocaine, amphetamine, methamphetamine & derivatives, OTC decongestants (phenylpropanolamine, ephedrine, pseudoephedrine). In caffeine/theophylline overdose, similar findings except for psychiatric signs results from catecholamine release.

Opiate, sedative, or ethanol intoxication
- Common signs: Coma, respiratory depression, miosis, hypotension, bradycardia, hypothermia, pulmonary edema, decreased bowel sounds, hyporeflexia, and needle marks. Seizures may occur after overdoses of some narcotics, notably propoxyphene.
- Common causes: Narcotics, barbiturates, benzodiazepines, ethchlorvynol, glutethimide, methprylon, methaqualone, meprobamate, ethanol, clonidine, & guanabenz.

Cholinergic syndromes
- Common signs: Confusion, CNS depression, weakness, emesis, salivation, lacrimation, urinary & fecal incontinence, GI cramping, emesis, diaphoresis, muscle fasciculation, pulmonary edema, miosis, bradycardia or tachycardia, seizures.
- Common causes: Organophosphate and carbamate insecticides, physostigmine, edrophonium, and some mushrooms.

---

[56] K Kulig, "Initial management of ingestions of toxic substances," N Engl J Med,1992;326(25):1677-81. Reprinted with permission of *The New England Journal of Medicine*, Copyright 1992,c Massachusetts Medical Society

Poisoning: Salicylate[57]

Mechanisms
- Central respiratory stimulation causes hyperventilation, respiratory alkalosis & compensatory metabolic acidosis leading to dehydration • Uncouples oxidative phosphorylation, inhibits Krebs cycle →lactic acidosis. • Hepatic damage causes coagulopathy. • Causes cerebral & pulmonary edema, unknown mechanism.

Presentation
- Dose > 160 mg/kg considered toxic.
- **Acute**: Vomiting, tachypnea, tinnitus, lethargy with ABG changes noted above. Severe: coma, seizures, hypoglycemia, pyrexia, pulmonary edema. Death from cerebral edema & cardiovascular collapse. Toxicity predicted from nomogram below. Measure **serial levels**: delayed absorption is common.
- **Chronic**: Young children & confused elderly. Nonspecific confusion, dehydration, metabolic acidosis. Cerebral & pulmonary edema more common than acute. Toxicity correlates poorly with levels.

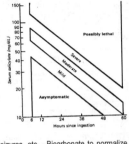

Treatment
- Supportive care for pulmonary failure, seizures, etc. • Bicarbonate to normalize pH. • Judicious fluid replacement in light of possible pulmonary edema. • Activated charcoal & cathartic in high-doses. • Urinary alkalinization (pH > 8) enhances elimination. • Hemodialysis for acute intoxociation & levels > 120 mg/dL, chronic & levels > 60 mg/dL, or any pt with severe toxicity. • Observe for prolonged period if enteric release tablets (may be visible on CXR).

Poisoning: Tricyclic Antidepressants[58]

Physiologic Toxicity
- Class 1a antiarrhythmic effects (prolong QRS and QT) • Induce catecholamine release and block reuptake • Anticholinergic activity • α-adrenergic antagonism

Clinical manifestations
- Altered sensorium. Anticholinergic effects: delirium, mydriasis, gastric atony • Coma • Seizure • QRS widening • Ventricular arrhythmia • Hypotension • Tachycardia

ECG signs[59]
- R in aV_R > 3 mm (0.3 mV) • Terminal 40mS of QRS has rightward axis • QRS duration > 110 mS • Resting tachycardia • QTc > 440 mS

Triage
- Altered sensorium warrants aggressive treatment and ICU monitoring[60]
- Asymptomatic patients 6 hours post-ingestion unlikely to suffer toxicity[61].

[57] JL Rippe et al (eds) Intensive Care Medicine, 2/e, Boston: Little-Brown, 1991.
[58] Cummins RO (ed.), American Heart Association, Textbook of Advanced Cardiac Life Support, Dallas: AHA, 1994, pp 10.19-10.20. Frommer DA, et al, "Tricyclic antidepressant overdose. A review," Jama, 1987;257(4):521-6.
[59] Liebelt EL, et al, "ECG lead aVR versus QRS interval in predicting seizures and arrhythmias in acute tricyclic antidepressant toxicity," Ann Emerg Med, 1995;26(2):195-201. Niemann JT, et al, "Electrocardiographic criteria for tricyclic antidepressant cardiotoxicity," Am J Cardiol, 1986;57(13):1154-9.
[60] Emerman CL, et al, "Level of consciousness as a predictor of complications following tricyclic overdose," Ann Emerg Med, 1987;16(3):326-30.
[61] Callaham M, Kassel D, "Epidemiology of fatal tricyclic antidepressant ingestion: implications for management," Ann Emerg Med, 1985; 14(1):1-9.

Management goals

- **Decontamination** with orogastric lavage and/or charcoal.
- **Alkalinization** shifts TCA → serum protein binding, counteracts Na-channel blockade. **Sodium bicarbonate** indicated in any hemodynamic instability, seizure, or ECG alteration above. Goal pH 7.50-7.55. Bolus 1 mEq/kg bicarbonate followed by "normal bicarbonate" (3×50mEq ampules in 1L D5W) at least 200 mL/hr infusion until ECG abnormalities reverse. Recheck pH often.
- **Magnesium** sulfate for long-QT arrhythmias (*Torsades de Pointes*) 2g bolus.
- **Hyperventilation** for seizing or arresting patients, to raise pH>7.50.

Seizures → acidosis which liberates protein-bound TCA, exacerbating toxicity
Hypotension usually responds to volume. Bicarbonate or vasopressors for nonresponders.

Cardiac arrest

- **PEA:** Hyperventilation, Bicarbonate to pH>7.5, Saline. Epinephrine if no prompt response. Consider other causes.
- **Ventricular arrhythmias:** Lidocaine followed by infusion if patient responds; otherwise IV Magnesium. Refractory VT may respond to phenytoin. **Avoid procainamide** which also is a Class 1a antiarrhythmic.
- **Ventricular fibrillation:** Defibrillate × 3 → Intubate → Epinephrine → Alkalinize/Hyperventilate → Lidocaine/Magnesium/Bretylium

Poisoning: Acetaminophen

Rumack-Matthew nomogram[62]

Note time of ingestion may be difficult to determine; treat aggressively.

Hepatic toxicity[63]

Primary toxic metabolite produced by cytochrome P450, ↑ed by ethanol, phenytoin, zidovudine. Alcoholics may have depleted glutathione stores. Severe hepatitis or fulminant hepatic failure may occur after single doses of 7.5-15g in normal adults or less than 4g in alcoholics[64]; great interindividual variability.

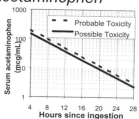

Therapy: See acetylcysteine (p 94).

---

[62] BH Rumack & H Matthew, "Acetaminophen poisoning and toxicity," Pediatrics, 1975:55(6):871-6.

[63] Vale JA, Proudfoot AT, "Paracetamol (acetaminophen) poisoning," Lancet 1995;346(8974):547-552.

[64] Zimmerman HJ, Maddrey WC, "Acetaminophen (paracetamol) hepatotoxicity with regular intake of alcohol: analysis of instances of therapeutic misadventure," Hepatology 1995;22(3):767-73.

Cardiology

Perioperative Cardiac Risk

Goals
- Identify high risk patients → delay elective surgery, consider for preoperative revascularization or special perioperative care.
- Identify low risk patients → proceed with surgery.
- Intermediate risk pts → stratify as high- or low-risk based eg on stress testing
- Coronary cath & revascularization (PTCA, CABG) if indicated apart from surgery

Goldman[65] and Detsky[66] modified cardiac risk indices

	Goldman	Points	Detsky	Points
Age	> 70 yo	5	> 70 yo	5
Coronary disease	MI within 6 mo	10	MI within 6 mo	10
			MI > 6 mo ago	5
			CCS angina class III	10
			CCS angina class IV	20
			Unstable angina past 3 mo	10
CHF	S3 or JVD	11	Pulm edema within 1 wk	10
			Pulm edema, ever	5
Rhythm	Other than NSR/PACs on most recent ECG	7	Other than NSR/PACs on last preop ECG	5
	> 5 PVCs/min any time preop	7	> 5 PVCs/min any time preop	5
Valvular disease	Important aortic stenosis	5	Suspected critical AS	20
General medical condition	P_aO_2<60 or P_aCO_2 >50, K <3.0 or HCO_3<20, BUN>50 or Cr>3.0, abnl AST, signs of chronic liver dz, bedridden from noncardiac causes	3	P_aO_2<60 or P_aCO_2 >50, K <3.0 or HCO_3<20, BUN>50 or Cr>3.0, abnl AST, signs of chronic liver dz, bedridden from noncardiac causes	5
Surgery	Intraperitoneal, thoracic, aortic surgery	3	Emergency surgery	10
	Emergency surgery	4		

Risk groups
Pooled odds ratios of perioperative MI, pulmonary edema, VT, cardiac death.

Class	Goldman points	odds[67]	Detsky points	odds[68]
I	0-5	0.29	0-15	0.42
II	6-12	0.94	16-30	3.58
III	13-25	3.4	>30	14.93
IV	≥ 26	22.7		

[65] Goldman et al, "Multifactorial index of cardiac risk in noncardiac surgical procedures," N Engl J Med 1977;297:845-50.
[66] Detsky AS, et al, "Predicting cardiac complications in patients undergoing noncardiac surgery," J Gen Intern Med 1986;1:211-9.
[67] L Goldman & E Braunwald, "General anesthesia and noncardiac surgery in patients with heart disease," in E Braunwald (ed) Heart Disease, Philadelphia: Saunders, 1992, p 1717.
[68] Detsky AS, et al, "Cardiac assessment for patients undergoing noncardiac surgery: a mutifactorial clinical risk index," Arch Intern Med, 1986; 146(11):2131-4.

Risk of major complications according to class & operation[69]

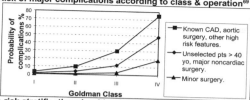

Probability of complications %

Goldman Class

- ■ Known CAD, aortic surgery, other high risk features.
- ◆ Unselected pts > 40 yo, major noncardiac surgery.
- ▲ Minor surgery.

A risk stratification algorithm for peripheral vascular surgery[70]

- **Intermediate risk** patients → Pharmacologic stress-imaging test; either
  (a) Goldman < 12 points and one or two **Eagle criteria**:
  (age>70; DM; angina; ECG Q waves; hx ventricular arrhythmia);
  (b) Cannot walk 2 blocks at normal pace without angina
  May not be superior to age>65 or hx of CAD in risk assessment
- **High risk** if **(a)** Goldman > 12 points; **(b)** Eagle > 2 criteria; **(c)** "Ischemia" on stress-imaging test; **(d)** Ischemia on rest or ambulatory ECG

Interventions to reduce perioperative cardiac complications

- Perioperative β-blockers may reduce long-term morbidity & mortality[71] (eg atenolol 5-10 mg IV over 5-10 min as long as HR>55 and SBP>100, given 30 minutes preop and immediately postop followed by 50-100mg po qd).
- Nitrates and Ca-blockers probably have limited benefit.
- Aspirin if acceptable to surgeons.
- Avoid negative inotropes in severe LV dysfunction (ie consider spinal or opiate-based anesthesia).
- Hemodynamic monitoring (PA catheter, ? continuous 12-lead ECG, ? TEE) in **(a)** MI in past 6 wks without revascularization **(b)** large unrevascularized myocardial territory; **(c)** severe LV dysfunction; **(d)** severe aortic or mitral valve disease; **(e)** aortic cross-clamping; **(f)** emergency surgery without optimized hemodynamics.
- Scrupulous postoperative BP, pain, volume management.

69 DT Mangano, L Goldman, "Preoperative assessment of patients with known or suspected coronary artery disease," N Engl J Med 1995; 333: 146(11):2131-4.. Reprinted by permission of *The New England Journal of Medicine*, Copyright 1995, Massachusetts Medical Society.
70 Wong T, Detsky AS, "Preoperative cardiac risk assessment for patients having periph vasc surgery," Ann Intern Med 1992;116(9):743. Eagle KA, et al, "Combining clinical and thallium data optimizes preoperative assessment of cardiac risk before major vascular surgery," Ann Intern Med, 1989;110:859. JB Baron et al, "Dipyridamole-thallium scintigraphy and gated radionuclide angiography to assess cardiac risk before abdominal aortic surgery," N Engl J Med, 1994; 330:663. Raby KE, et al, "Correlation between preoperative ischemia and major cardiac events after peripheral vascular surgery," N Engl J Med, 1989; 321:1296
71 Mangano DT, et al, "Effect of atenolol on mortality after cardiovascular morbidity after noncardiac surgery," N Engl J Med 1996; 335(23):1713-20.

Probability of Coronary Disease[72]

Likelihood of significant coronary disease based on history

Sex/Age	Asymptomatic	Non-Anginal	Atypical angina	Typical Angina
Men				
60-69	.12	.28	.67	.94
50-59	.10	.22	.59	.92
40-49	.06	.14	.46	.87
30-39	.02	.05	.22	.70
Women				
60-69	.08	.19	.54	.91
50-59	.03	.08	.32	.79
40-49	.01	.03	.13	.55
30-39	.00	.01	.04	.26

Post-exercise test probability of significant CAD

Age Sex	Asymptomatic		Non-Anginal		Atypical Angina		Typical Angina	
	M	F	M	F	M	F	M	F
ST depression > 2.5 mm								
30-39	43±25	11±9	68±22	24±20	92±8	98±2	99±1	93±7
40-49	69±21	28±21	87±12	53±26	97±3	95±5	100±.4	98±2
50-59	81±16	56±25	91±8	78±17	98±2	86±13	100±.2	99±.7
60-69	96±13	76±18	94±6	90±9	99±1	63±25	100±.2	100±.3
ST depression 2-2.5 mm								
30-39	18±10	3±2	38±17	8±6	76±13	93±5	96±3	79±13
40-49	39±17	10±7	65±16	24±14	91±6	84±9	98±1	93±5
50-59	54±17	27±14	75±13	50±18	94±4	63±17	99±.5	98±2
60-69	61±16	47±17	81±11	72±14	96±3	33±17	100±.4	99±.6
ST depression 1.5-2.0 mm								
30-39	8±5	1±1	19±11	3±2.5	55±18	16±10	91±6	59±19
40-49	20±11	4±3	41±17	11±7.2	78±12	39±18	97±2	84±10
50-59	31±15	12±8	53±18	28±14	86±9	67±16	98±1	94±4
60-69	37±16	25±13	62±17	49±18	90±7	83±10	99±1	98±2
ST depression 1.0-1.5								
30-39	4±1	.6±.2	10±2	2±.7	38±5	50±5	83±3	42±9
40-49	11±2	2±.5	26±4	6±2	64±4	72±4	94±1	72±6
50-59	19±2.6	7±1	37±5	16±3	75±3	9±3	96±.7	89±2
60-69	23±3	15±2	45±5	33±5	81±3	25±6	97±.5	95±1
ST depression 0.5-1.0								
30-39	2±.6	.3±.1	5±2	.7±.4	21±6	52±8	68±7	24±8
40-49	5±2	1±.3	13±4	3±1	44±8	4±2	86±4	53±10
50-59	9±3	3±1	20±5	8±2	57±8	31±7	91±3	78±6
60-69	11±3	7±2	26±6	17±5	65±7	12±4	94±2	95±1

[72] GA Diamond, JS Forrester, "Analysis of probability as an aid in the clinical diagnosis of coronary artery disease," N Engl J Med, 1979;300:1350. Reprinted by permission of The New England Journal of Medicine, Copyright 1979, Massachusetts Medical Society.

Exercise Stress Testing

Objectives of exercise testing

• **Diagnosing coronary disease**, or identifying patients likely to have functionally-significant coronary obstruction. • Evaluating **functional capacity**, as opposed to simple anatomic abnormalities: Need for medical or surgical therapy; Adequacy of medical or surgical therapy; Safety of work or recreation • Estimating **prognosis** in patients with known coronary disease, identifying patients who need more definitive therapy

Limitations of Exercise Tests in detecting coronary disease

• Limited or no value in certain common situations: **Women**: High false-positive rate (ST segment response); Positive tests do not add much to predictive value of H&P alone. **Beta-blockers** therapeutic effect limits maximum work (heart rate x blood pressure), thereby decreasing sensitivity. **Digitalis** depresses ST segments, usually not more than 0.1 mV. Further exertional ST-depression usually reflects ischemia. Consider stopping dig > one week before test; **Conduction abnormalities (BBB, Preexcitation)** cause abnormal sequence of activation and repolarization making ST segments uninterpretable (except lateral precordial leads in RBBB). **(e) Pressure overload (LVH, Aortic Stenosis)** causes subendocardial ischemia and ST depression even in absence of CAD. True-positive test for ischemia; false-positives for epicardial coronary obstruction.
• The patient has to be **able to exercise**.
• **Uncertainty** about whether the patient has an anatomic abnormality.

ACC/AHA Indications for Exercise Testing[73]

Suspected or known coronary artery disease (CAD)
Class I (Generally accepted)
 • Help diagnose CAD in men with **atypical** symptoms of ischemia
 • Assess **prognosis** and **functional capacity** in pts with known CAD
 • To evaluate suspected recurrent **exercise-induced dysrhythmias**
Class II (Controversial)
 To help diagnose CAD in **Women** with typical or atypical symptoms of ischemia; Patients taking **digitalis** or with **RBBB**. Evaluate **drug tx and functional capacity** in pts with CAD/CHF. To evaluate **variant angina**. Serial evaluation of patients with **known CAD.**
Class III (No justification)
 • Diagnosing CAD in patients with **preexcitation** or **LBBB**. Evaluation of single **PVC's** without evidence of CAD. Evaluating serially in course of exercise **cardiac rehabilitation**

Screening of apparently healthy individuals

Class I (Generally accepted) : None
Class II (Controversial): Asymptomatic men over age 40 with risky jobs: pilots, bus drivers. Asymptomatic men with at least two known CAD risks (chol > 240, HTN, tobacco, DM, family hx CAD < 55yrs). Sedentary men over age 40 entering vigorous exercise.
Class III: Asymptomatic men and women without known risks. Evaluation of clinically "noncardiac" chest pain.

After myocardial infarction

Class I (Generally accepted) : To evaluate after CABG or PTCA
Class II: (Controversial) Yearly asymptomatic patients after CABG/PTCA

Valvular heart disease

Class I: None;   Class II (Controversial): Functional capacity;
Class III: Evaluate symptomatic critical AS or hypertrophic cardiomyopathy

[73] RC Schlant, et al, "Guidelines for exercise testing," J Am Coll Cardiol 1986;8(3):725-38.

Hypertension
Class I (Generally accepted): None; Class II: BP response in HTN for pts who wish to exercise vigorously; Class III: Severe HTN, HTN not wishing exercise

Exercise testing with thallium perfusion scintigraphy
- Modest ↑ in sensitivity and specificity for CAD compared to EST alone
- Helpful when expected likelihood of CAD is intermediate; conversely **unlikely to help** when suspicion of CAD is low or high
- Preferable to EST without thallium in patients with abnormal resting ECG (generally similar specificity but lower sensitivity)

The Duke Prognostic Score[74]

Score =	(Exercise duration, min) — (5 × max ST-deviation, mm) — (4 × treadmill angina index)

Treadmill angina index: 0 = None; 1 = Nonlimiting angina; 2 = Angina stops test

Risk of death	Inpatients	4-yr Survival	Outpatients	4-yr Survival
Low (≥ +5)	470 (34%)	0.98	379 (62%)	0.99
Mod (-10 to +4)	795 (57%)	0.92	211 (34%)	0.95
High (< -10)	129 (9%)	0.71±0.06	23 (4%)	0.79±0.11

ECG — Hypertrophy[75]

Left Ventricular Hypertrophy (Romhilt-Estes criteria)

Limb lead R or S amplitude > 2.0mV or S in V1 or V2 > 3.0mV or R in V5 or V6 > 3.0mV	3 points	Total Points: 4 : LVH likely 5 : LVH present
ST segment abnormality: Without digitalis	2 points	
With digitalis	1 point	
Left atrial enlargement	3 points	**Sensitivity 50%**
Left axis deviation > -30	2 points	**Specificity 95%**
QRS duration > 0.09sec	1 point	
Intrinsicoid deflection V5 and V6 > 0.05	1 point	

Left ventricular hypertrophy (Cornell criteria)[76]
- R (aVL) + S (V3) ≥ 2.8 mV (men), ≥ 2.0 mV (women)

Right Ventricular Hypertrophy (any of the following)
- RAXD > 100⁰ without AWMI, IWMI, LPFB, RBBB
- R in V1 >= 7mm.
- R > S in V1 (in absence of posterior MI).
- R < S in V5 or V6.
- RBBB with RAXD (in 1st 60mS of QRS) or R/S<2 in lead I
- rSR' complex in V1 with QRS duration < 120 mS (iRBBB)

Causes of dominant R in V1&V2[77]
Normal variant; RV hypertrophy; Posterior infarction; WPW; LV diastolic overload; Hypertrophic cardiomyopathy; Duchenne's muscular dystrophy

[74] DB Mark, *et al*, "Prognostic value of exercise score in outpatients with suspected coronary artery disease," N Engl J Med, 1991;325(12):849.
[75] Romhilt et al, "A critical appraisal of the ECG criteria for the diagnosis of left ventricular hypertrophy," Circulation 1969;40:185.
[76] Casale PN *et al*," Circulation, 1987;75(3):565-72.
[77] HJL Marriot, Practical electrocardiography, 8/e, Baltimore: Williams & Wilkins, 1988, p55.

ECG Wide-Complex Tachycardia[78]

Diagnosis of ventricular tachycardia

Inexact features suggestive of VT
- Extreme left axis deviation
- QRS duration > 140mS (RBBB morphology), >160mS (LBBB morph)
- "Fusion" complexes, in which atrial rhythm "captures" QRS
- QRS concordance in V leads (V leads all entirely positive or negative)
- Net area under QRS negative both in leads I and II

(Cumulative **Sensitivity/Specificity**)

Brugada criteria (any of the following, in stepwise fashion)
- RS absent in **all** precordial leads = VT ....21 / 1.0
  (May include QS, QR, monophasic R)
- R-S interval > 100 mS (onset of R to nadir of S) ⟶ 66/.98
  in **any** precordial leads = VT
- A-V dissociation = VT 82/.98
- Morphology criteria for VT **both leads V1-2 AND V6** 99/.98
  - RBBB - like QRS (predominantly positive in V1)

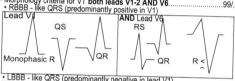

- LBBB - like QRS (predominantly negative in lead V1)

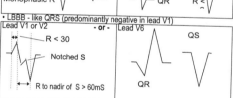

- Supraventricular tachycardia in absence of above conditions 97/.99
- **CLINICAL APPEARANCE DOES NOT DISTINGUISH SVT from VT!**

---

[78] Brugada et al, "A new approach to the differential diagnosis of a regular tachycardia with a wide QRS complex," Circulation 1991;83:1649-1659.; Note these patients were not taking antiarrhythmic drugs. Diagrams adapted from Tom Evans, MD, with permission.

ECG: BBB, Fascicle Block & IWMI[79]

Left bundle branch block

- QRS > 120 mS
- Abnormal septal activation R → L: <u>absent septal Q</u>
- Slow R → L activation: slurred R wave leads I & V_6
- Prominent delay <u>late</u> in QRS: notched R in I and V_6
- Individuals have unpredictable A-P & inferosuperior activation patterns:
  - Frontal axis may be normal or leftward
  - Right-precordial R waves may be present or absent
- Absent Q waves in LBBB obscure myocardial scar
- ST- and T-wave vector opposite to QRS vector; Isoelectric ST-segment and concordant T-waves may suggest myocardial ischemia
- Incomplete LBBB:
  - QRS 100-120 mS   • Loss of septal Q wave
  - Slurred/notched QRS in I and V_6

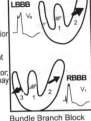

Bundle Branch Block

Right bundle branch block

- QRS > 120 mS   • Normal septal activation
- Terminal portion of QRS vector rightward and anterior:
  - V1: Initial R from normal septal activation; subsequent S from LV activation; terminal R' from delayed RV activation
  - I, V_5, V_6: Initial Q from normal septal activation, R from normal LV activation, prolonged shallow S wave from delayed RV activation
- T wave vector opposite the **terminal** portion of QRS
- Early activation intact: Q wave of myocardial scar is intact
- Incomplete RBBB:
  - QRS 100-120 mS   • Morphology criteria of RBBB (RsR' pattern in V_1, prolonged shallow S wave in lateral leads)

ECG —Left Anterior Fascicular Block

VCG: Frontal plane forces counterclockwise, initially inferior & terminally superior; therefore aVL peaks before aVR.
  (1) QRS complexes in $_aV_R$ and $_aV_L$ each end in an R wave, **and**
  (2) Peak of the terminal R wave in $_aV_R$ occurs later than the peak of terminal R wave in $_aV_L$.
Scalar criteria: QRS axis -45⁰ – -90⁰; QRS<120mS; Small Q in lead I; Small R in II, III, $_aV_F$; Late intrinsicoid deflection in $_aV_L$ (>45mS)

Left Posterior Fascicular Block

VCG: QR complex in II, III, $_aV_F$ from initial superior and final inferior force
Scalar criteria: QRS axis +90⁰; Initial R in I, $_aV_L$+ Small Q in II, III, $_aV_F$; QRS < 120 mS; Late intrinsicoid deflection in $_aV_F$ (>45mS); All **in absence of** pulmonary disease, vertical heart position, RVH, WPW.

Inferior Wall MI (Sensitivity & Specificity > 90%)

VCG: Initial frontal forces clockwise and superior
- Clockwise rotation of frontal plane (lead II peaks before lead III) and
  - Q waves > 30mS in lead II, **or**
  - Regression of initial inferior forces from lead III to lead II (initial portion of QRS is more negative in lead II than in lead III)

---

[79] RA Warner, "Recent advances in the diagnosis of myocardial infarction," Cardiology Clinics, 1987;5(3):381; RA Warner, et al, "Improved ECG criteria for the diagnosis of left anterior hemiblock," Am J Cardiol, 1983;51:723.

Inferior Wall MI + Left Anterior Fascicular Block (both of:)
(1) $_aV_R$ and $_aV_L$ both end in R waves; terminal R of $_aV_L$ before $_aV_R$; and
(2) Q of any magnitude in lead II
VCG: initial superior and clockwise; terminal superior and counterclockwise

AHA Permanent Pacing Indications[80]

Guidelines should also take into account
Good quality of life or prognosis; underlying cardiac disease that may be adversely affected by bradycardia; desire to drive a car; remoteness of medical care, including pts who live alone; medication that may depress escape heart rates or aggravate AVB; slowing of basic escape rates; significant cerebrovascular disease that might result in a stroke if cerebral perfusion were suddenly to decrease; desires of the patient and family

Permanent Pacing in acquired AV block in adults
Class I (Generally acceptable):
• Complete heart block associated with any of the following:
  • Symptomatic bradycardia. CHB is presumed cause of any symptoms unless specifically proven otherwise. • CHF • Conditions requiring medications that suppress automaticity of escape pacemakers and result in symptomatic bradycardia. • Documented asystole > 3.0s or asymptomatic escape rate <40bpm. • Confusional states that clear with temporary pacing. • Post AV junction ablation • Myotonic dystrophy
• Any second degree AVB, perm or intermit, with symptomatic brady.
• Afib, Aflutter, SVT with CHB or advanced AVB unrelated to nodal-blocking drugs and any of the conditions under CHB above.
Class II (Controversial):
• Asymptomatic CHB, perm or intermit, with ventricular rates > 40bpm.
• Asymptomatic Type II second-degree AVB, permanent or intermittent
• Asymptomatic Type I second-degree AVB at intra- or infra-His levels.
Class III (No justification):
• First degree AVB • Asymptomatic type I second-degree AVB at supra-His level.

Permanent Pacing after MI (not necessarily symptoms)
Class I (Generally acceptable): • Persistent advanced second degree AVB or CHB after acute MI with block in the His-Purkinje system (bilateral BBB)
• Transient advanced AVB and associated BBB.
Class II (Controversial): • Persistent advanced block at the AV node.
Class III (No justification): • Transient AV conduction disturbances in the absence of IVCD • Transient AVB in presence of LAHB • Acquired LAHB in absence of AVB • Persistent first-degree AVB in presence of (new) BBB.

Permanent pacing in bifascicular and trifascicular block (Rate of progression of bifascicular block to CHB is extremely low)
Class I (Generally acceptable)
• Bifascicular block with intermittent CHB associated with symptomatic brady.
• Bi- or trifascicular block with intermittent Type II second degree AVB without symptoms attributable to the heart block
Class II (Controversial):
• Bi- or trifascicular block with syncope that is not proved to be due to CHB, but other possible causes for syncope are not identifiable
• Markedly prolonged HV (>100mS)
• Pacing-induced infra-His block
Class III (No justification):
• Fascicular block with 1°AVB or (without AVB or symptoms)

---

[80] "Guidelines for implantation of cardiac pacemakers and antiarrhythmia devices," JACC 1991;18(1):1-13.

Permanent pacing in sinus node dysfunction

Class I (Generally acceptable) • Sinus node dysfunction with documented symptomatic bradycardia, including as a consequence of necessary drug tx.

Class II (Controversial) • Sinus node dysfunction, spontaneously or as a result of necessary drug therapy, with heart rates <40 when a clear association between significant symtpoms consistent with bradycardia and the actual presence of bradycardia has not been documented.

Class III (No justification) • Asymptomatic SND, including HR<40 as consequence of long-term drugs. • SND in whom symptoms suggestive of bradycardia are clearly documented not to be associated with a slow heart rate.

Pacing in hypersensitive carotid sinus & neurovascular syndromes (distinction between cardioinhibitory & vasodepressor response)

Class I • Recurrent syncope associated with clear, spontaneous events provoked by carotid sinus stimulation; minimal carotid sinus pressure induces asystole > 3s in the absence of sinus/AVN depressor medication.

Class II • Recurrent syncope without clear, provocative events and with a hypersensitive cardioinhibitory response. • Syncope with associated bradycardia reproduced by a head-up tilt with or without isoproterenol (or other provocations) and in which a temporary pacemaker and a second provocative test can establish the likely benefits of a permanent pacer.

Class III • Hyperactive cardioinhibitory response to carotid sinus stim without Sx • Vague Sx (dizziness, lightheadedness) with a hyperactive cardioinhibitory response to carotid sinus stimulation. • Recurrent syncope, light-headedness or dizziness in the absence of a cardioinhibitory response.

Emergency Cardiac Pacing

Indications: See "ACLS Emergency Cardiac Pacing" on page **16**.

Procedures

• Apply ECG leads before prep. Keep R+L arm leads or a V lead accessible.
• Usual sheath route R IJ or L subclavian. Scrupulous asepsis essential even in emergencies; catheter will probably remain for days.
• If fluoroscope unavailable: Balloon flotation in ventricle; J-wire for atrium.
• Insert while pt breathes deeply to drag balloon-tipped catheter into atrium.
• **"Injury current" technique:**
  • Attach distal (-, black) lead to V (chest) electrode of ECG. This will show a unipolar electrogram on the corresponding V lead. Or attach distal (-, black) electrode to R arm and proximal (+, red) electrode to L arm of ECG: Lead I yields bipolar, II & III unipolar electrograms.
  • Advance catheter with ECG running. QRS voltage increases as you enter the RV. Voltage decreases if you enter the IVC or PA. Suspect malposition if catheter exceeds 35 cm from R IJ approach.
  • Catheter trauma may precipitate VT; withdrawal usually stops it.
  • Deflate balloon and advance the catheter. An **injury current** (ST segment ↑ resembling MI) reflects endocardial contact. Advance ~1cm further to ensure good contact.
• **"Pace-capture" technique** (Used in true emergencies)
  • Advantages: simplicity/speed; Disadvantages: ↓ safety.
  • Attach leads to pacemaker generator. Monitor ECG. Turn generator ON: rate 70-100 bpm, output max, sensitivity 0/demand.
  • Advance pacing catheter until ventricle is successfully captured.
• After placement, leave balloon deflated and test thresholds (see below).

Threshold testing

• **Pacing** (stimulation) **threshold**: minimum energy for successful capture.

- Set pacing rate higher than intrinsic heart rate
- Set generator at maximum output; note succesful capture. Otherwise check for stimulus artifact on ECG, battery (output lamp), connections, placement, consider myocardial unresponsiveness (eg, acidosis).
- Monitor ECG, gradually ↓ pacemaker output (mA) until capture fails, at the *stimulation threshold*. If > 2 mA may reflect unreliable placement.
- Set output to 1.5-3-times threshold. Maximum output setting more reliable but may also increase risk of VF.
- **Sensing** (inhibition) **threshold**: detected voltage which inhibits pacing, eg when intrinsic heart rate is adequate.
- Proper sensing permits pacer inhibition by normal QRSs but not T waves and other noise. Also avoids pacing during repolarization (R-on-T phenomenon) which can induce VF. Terminology is confusing:
  - "High sensitivity" = little energy required to inhibit the pacemaker; "Low sensitivity" = much energy required.
  - "Demand" = highest sensitivity: detection of minimal energy will inhibit pacer, including artifact like muscle movement or T waves.
  - "Async" = lowest sensitivity: pacemaker will fire even though it detects much energy, eg from the QRS complex.
- Set pacemaker rate to below intrinsic heart rate (if that rate is hemodynamically unacceptable, abort test).
- Begin with sensitivity set at 0 or "demand;" this should inhibit pacing. With real-time ECG monitoring, gradually decrease sensitivity until the pacemaker fires appropriately (whenever the heart rate falls below the set rate). This is the *sensitivity threshold*, usually 0.5-2mA.
- Set sensitivity to approximately 1.3-2 times the threshold, but check to make sure the device is not inhibited by artifacts like T waves. Some believe emergency pacemakers should be set in "demand" mode.

Intraaortic balloon pump

Indications
- Myocardial ischemia: refractory unstable angina or postinfarction angina; refractory polymorphic VT; support for PTCA
- Cardiogenic shock: Pump failure; Acute mitral regurgitation or acute ventricular septal rupture as a bridge to definitive tx
- Postoperative myocardial depression and weaning from bypass

Contraindications
- No definitive treatment available for underlying pathology; • Moderate-severe aortic insufficiency; • Severe aortic or iliofemoral vascular dz;

Operating the IABP
- <u>Balloon deflation</u> • Nadir of end-diastolic pressure just before arterial upstroke (aortic valve opening) begins • Late deflation: ventricle contracts against inflated balloon • Premature deflation: suboptimal afterload reduction
- <u>Balloon inflation</u> • Just after dicrotic notch • Early inflation: ventricle contracts against inflated balloon • Late inflation: excessive diastolic hypotension, suboptimal augmentation of coronary flow
- Full anticoagulation

Complications
- Leg ischemia • Aortic dissection • femoral or retroperitoneal hemorrhage • Pseudoaneurysm • Infection • Thromboembolism • ↓ Platelets • Lymph obstruction

Timing examples[81]: Arterial pressure waveforms with 1:2 counterpulsation.

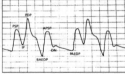

Correct timing. Balloon aortic end-diastolic
pressure (BAEDP) is lower than aortic
end-diastolic pressure (PAEDP). Assisted
peak systolic pressure (APSP) is lower
than native peak systolic pressure (PSP).
IP = inflation point.

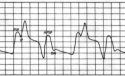

Early inflation. Inflation point (IP) occurs
before aortic valve closure, before dicrotic
notch (DN).

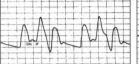

Late inflation. IP occurs after DN with
shortening of diastolic augmentation time
and small augmented waveform.

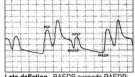

Late deflation. BAEDP exceeds PAEDP;
it should be lower.

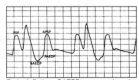

Early deflation. BAEDP occurs early and
equilibrates rapidly with nonaugmented
PAEDP; augmented peak systolic
pressure (APSP) is improperly higher than
nonaugmented PSP.

[81] M Sorrentino, T Feldman, "Techniques for IABP timing, use, and discontinuance," J Critical Illness,
1992;7(4):597-604, with permission of Cliggott Publishing.

Coronary Artery Anatomy[82]

LEFT CORONARY ARTERY

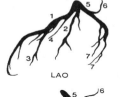

LAO

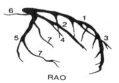

RAO

LAO-CRANIAL ANGULATION

1. LEFT ANTERIOR DESCENDING ARTERY WITH SEPTAL BRANCHES
2. RAMUS MEDIANUS
3. DIAGONAL ARTERY
4. FIRST SEPTAL BRANCH
5. LEFT CIRCUMFLEX ARTERY
6. LEFT ATRIAL CIRCUMFLEX ARTERY
7. OBTUSE MARGINAL ARTERY

RIGHT CORONARY ARTERY

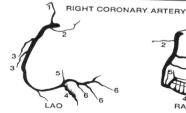

LAO

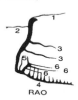

RAO

1. CONUS ARTERY
2. S-A NODE ARTERY
3. ACUTE MARGINAL ARTERY
4. POSTERIOR DESCENDING ARTERY WITH SEPTAL BRANCHES
5. A-V NODE ARTERY
6. POSTERIOR LEFT VENTRICULAR ARTERY

[82] From WG Grossman, Cardiac catheterization and angiography., 4th edition, Philadelphia: Lea and Febiger, 1991. Reproduced with permission.

Hemodynamics — Cardiac Cycle[83]

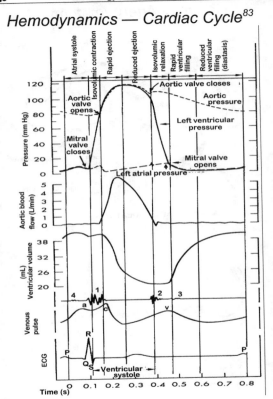

[83] Berne RM & Levy MN, <u>Cardiovascular Physiology</u>, 6th, St. Louis: Mosby, 1986, figure 3-13, with permission.

Jugular Venous Pulsations[84]

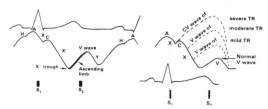

Systolic Murmurs[85]

Maneuver	Response	Sensitivity	Specificity	Positive Predictive Value	Negative Predictive Value
Right-sided murmurs					
Inspiration	Increase	100	88	67	100
Expiration	Decrease	100	88	67	100
Müller maneuver	Increase	15	92	33	81
Hypertrophic Cardiomyopathy					
Valsalva	Increase	65	96	81	92
Squatting to Standing	Increase	95	84	59	98
Standing to Squatting	Decrease	95	85	61	99
Leg elevation	Decrease	85	91	71	96
Handgrip	Decrease	85	75	46	95
Mitral regurgitation & VSD					
Handgrip	Increase	68	92	84	81
Transient arterial occlusion	Increase	78	100	100	87
Amyl nitrite inhalation	Decrease	80	90	84	87

- Aortic stenosis diagnosed by exclusion.
- Inspiration & Expiration: Patient breathed following listener's arm signal
- Müller maneuver: Occlude nares; Suck manometer (-)40-50 mmHg × 10s
- Valsalva: Exhale into manometer (+)490 mm Hg. Listen at end of strain phase.
- Squatting to standing: Squat 30s then rapidly stand. Listen first 15-20s standing.
- Standing to squatting: Avoid Valsalva. Listen immediately after squatting.
- Passive leg elevation: Pt supine, elevate 45 degrees. Listen 15-20s later.
- Isometric handgrip: Hand dynamometer, listen after one minute max contraction.
- Transient arterial occlusion: Sphygmo cuffs on both arms inflated 20-40 mm above systolic. Listen 20s later.
- Amyl nitrite: 0.3ml ampule broken, 3 rapid deep breaths. Listen 15-30s later.

[84] J Constant, Bedside Cardiology, 3rd, Boston: Little, Brown, 1985, pp95, 105. Published by Little, Brown and Company. Reproduced with permission.
[85] Lembo, et al, "Bedside diagnosis of systolic murmurs," N Engl J Med 1988; 318:1572-8. Reprinted with permission of The New England Journal of Medicine, Copyright 1988, Massachusetts Medical Society.

Selected characteristics of common systolic heart murmurs[86].

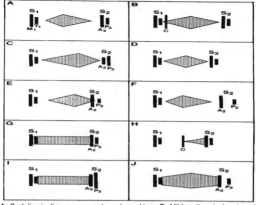

A: Systolic ejection murmur, note early peaking. **B:** Mild aortic valvular stenosis; note relatively early peaking and systolic ejection click. **C:** Severe aortic stenosis; note late peaking and decreased intensity of A_2. **D:** Hypertrophic cardiomyopathy. **E:** Severe pulmonary valvular stenosis; note late peaking with murmur extending through A_2 and delayed appearance of P_2. **F:** Atrial septal defect; note wide splitting of S_2. **G:** Uncomplicated mitral regurgitation; note holosystolic murmur extending through A_2. **H:** Mitral valve prolapse; note late systolic murmur ushered in by midsystolic click. **I:** Tricuspid regurgitation due to pulmonary hypertension; note holosystolic murmur beginning with T_1 and early, loud P_2. **J:** Uncomplicated ventricular septal defect; note loud, holosystolic murmur with midsystolic accentuation and slightly delayed P_2.

Long QT syndromes & Torsades[87]

Pause-Dependent
- **Drugs** (effect often dose-dependent): <u>Antiarrhythmics</u>: IA (quinidine, procainamide, disopyramide), III (amiodarone, sotalol esp in women, ? bretylium), bepridil, **not IC** agents • <u>Combinations</u>: *eg* (erythromycin or clarithomycin or troleandomycin or ketoconazole or itraconazole) and (terfenadine or astemizole) • <u>Tricyclic</u> & tetracyclic antiarrhythmics • <u>Phenothiazines</u> and butyrophenones • ? <u>Serotonergics</u> (ketanserin) • <u>Antimicrobials</u>: pentamidine, erythromycin, trimethaprim/sulfa • <u>Vasopressin</u> • <u>Organophosphage</u> insecticides

[86] MA Alpert, "Systolic murmurs," in HK Walker *et al*, (eds), <u>Clinical Methods</u>, pp 131-137, Boston: Butterworth-Heineman, 1991, adapted with permission.
[87] WM Jackman, *et al*, "Long QT syndromes: a critical review, new clinical observations, and a unifying hypothesis," <u>Progr Cardiovasc Dis</u> 31(2):115-172, 1988.

- **Electrolytes**: • hypokalemia, • hypomagnesemia
- **Nutrition**: • starvation, • anorexia nervosa, • liquid protein diet
- **Severe bradycardia**: • complete AVB, • sinus node dysfunction

Acute therapy options:
- Washout offending drug while monitoring • Correct electrolyte disorder
- Overdrive pacing 90-110 bpm • Magnesium sulfate 1-2 gm IV
- Isoproterenol gtt to keep ventricular rate > 90 bpm, caution in CAD
- Atropine 0.03 mg/kg IV in drug-induced TdP unrelated to AV block
- ? Bretylium may counteract QT prolongation from IA antiarrhythmics

Catecholamine-dependent
- **Congenital**   • **Sporadic**
  - Jervell & Lange-Nielson syndrome: congenital deafness, autosomal recessive inheritance). Seen ~ 0.2% congenital deaf children.
  - Romano-Ward syndrome: nl hearing, autosomal dominant, HLA A9bw
- **Atypical**: subarachnoid hemorrhage, stroke
? Autonomic manipulation by surgery: carotid endarterectomy, right radical neck dissection, transabdominal truncal vagotomy

Chronic therapy options:
- Beta-adrenergic blockade • AICD, pacing • Sympathectomy

Syncope
Differential diagnosis √ = dx by history/physical/ECG
⊗ = special tests (eg Holter, Tilt-table, invasive EP study, EEG, Carotid U/S)
- **#1 Cause: Idiopathic, undiagnosible, and/or benign syncope.**
- **Cardiac causes**
  - Reflex / autonomic
    - Situational/vasovagal
      √ Micturition/deglutition/defecation/postprandial/cough/Valsalva/ sneeze/oculovagal/Jacuzzi/diving/wt-lifting/late-pregnancy-supine
      ⊗ "Neurocardiogenic syncope"
      - Vasodepressor: vasodilation & inappropriate bradycardia. Setting of fear, emotion, pain, premonitory sx. Blocked by EPI. Stimulation of inferior-cardiac C-fibers (Bezold-Jarisch reflex).
      - Cardioinhibitory (frequent: AV block, prevented with atropine)
      √ Carotid sinus hypersensitivity (AV block on CS massage)
      √ Glossopharyngeal neuralgia (dysautonomia s/p neck surgery, RTX)
    - Orthostatic
      √ Drugs; √ Hyperadrenergic (eg Volume depletion / hemorrhage)
      √ Autonomic dz: Drugs; Neuropathy of DM or EtOH; Bedrest/deconditioning; Shy-Drager; Parkinson; B12 deficiency; Tabes
  - Electrical
    ⊗ Atrioventricular block → profound bradycardia (Stokes-Adams attack)
    ⊗Sinus node dysfunction (sick-sinus-syndrome); √ Pacemaker failure
    ⊗ Ventricular arrhythmias (VT, Torsades de Pointes, ?WPW, **not** VF)
    √ Long QT syndromes
    - Pause-dependent: drugs, electrolytes, stroke, carotid manipulation
    - Catecholamine-dependent: Romano-Ward, Lange-Jervell-Nielsen
    ⊗ Supraventricular arrhythmias
  - Mechanical
    √ Valvular/subvalvular obstruction: AS, MS, atrial myxoma, HCM/IHSS
    √ Pulmonary embolism / pulmonary hypetension

- **Noncardiac**
  - Neurologic: √ Primary seizure disorder; √ Vertebrobasilar insufficiency ("Drop attacks"): TIA; Subclavian steal; √ Takayasu; √ Arnold-Chiari malformation
  √ Metabolic: hypoglycemia, hypoxia, hyperventilation
  - Psychiatric: √ Panic disorder/hyperventilation; √ Hysteria

Drugs commonly causing postural hypotension & syncope

Vasodilators: hydralazine, minoxidil, nifedipine, nitrates, bretylium; α- and β-adrenergic blockers; *Diuretics*; *Antiarrhythmics* (Torsades); *Phenothiazines*; *Antidepressants*; *L-dopa*; *Vinca* alkaloids (autonomic neuropathy); *Insulin* (hypoglycemia)

Kapoor's experience of 433 patients[88]

Noncardiac		Cardiac	
Vasodepressor	35	Ventricular tachycardia	49
Situational	36	Sinus node dysfunction (SSS)	15
Drug-induced	9	Bradycardia	4
Orthostatic	43	Supraventricular tachycardia	8
TIA	8	Complete heart block	6
Subclavian Steal	2	Mobitz II A-V block	2
Seizure disorder	7	Pacemaker malfunction	3
Trigeminal neuralgia	1	Carotid sinus hypersensitivity	5
Conversion reaction	3	Aortic stenosis	8
		Myocardial infarction	5
		Aortic dissection	1
		Pulmonary thromboembolism	2
		Pulmonary hypertension	2
Total	144	Total	110

Unknown cause: 179

5-year Mortality:

	All-cause mortality	Sudden-death
Cardiac syncope	50%	30%
Noncardiac syncope	25%	5%
Syncope without identifiable cause	20%	<5%

Pearls & Nonsense

- Convulsions, loss of consciousness, trauma do not help identify etiology
- Exclude VT (structural heart disease) before attributing syncope to bradycardia.
- Postical state or Todd's paralysis suggests seizure as etiology
- CT, EEG, Carotid U/S don't identify CNS disease inapparent from H&P
- TIAs from carotid disease almost never cause syncope
- Head-up tilt-table exams are nonspecific for identifying vasovagal/vasodepressor syncope, especially when using isoproterenol

Laboratory tests in evaluation of syncope

- Identify risk of sudden death
  - If CAD + LV dysfunction → cath/revascularize; if revascularized then EP testing for inducible VT. Note (1) signal-averaged ECG predicts (+) EP test and (2) Good prognosis if EP unable to induce malignant arrythmia
- Identify paroxysmal rhythm disorders if routine evaluation is unrevealing
  - Telemetry if coronary disease or LV dysfunction
  - Holter monitor (with diary), event monitor, continuous loop monitor if no structural heart disease or telemetry is unrevealing

[88] WN Kapoor, "Evaluation and Outcome of Patients with Syncope," <u>Medicine</u>, 69(3):160-75, 1990. Copyright 1990 Waverly, With permission.

- EP testing is insensitive in reproducing culprit bradyarrhythmias
- Reserve expensive screening tests for recurrent syncope:
  eg head-up tilt-table testing; EEG
- Reserve neurological evaluation for pts with CNS complaints/findings

Endocrinology

Myxedema coma[89]

Precipitants: Stroke, hypothermia, infection, CHF, drugs (anesthetics, sedatives, tranquilizers, narcotics, lithium, amiodarone), trauma, GI bleed, concurrent metabolic disturbances ($\downarrow$ glucose, $\downarrow$ Na, $\uparrow$ CO_2, acidosis)

Features: (Hypothermia, ΔMS, identifiable precipitant) confer >50% mortality
- **Hypothermia** • **CNS:** Lethargy→stupor→coma; hastened by drugs; proceeds to resp failure; "myxedema madness:" depression, paranoia, hallucinations
- **Respiratory:** $\downarrow$ hypoxic and hypercapnic drive → hypoventilation; pleural effusions; airway obstruction from macroglossia & myxedema infiltrate • **Cardiac:** $\uparrow$ silhouette; bradycardia; $\downarrow$ heart sounds; ECG block, $\downarrow$ voltage, $\uparrow$ QT; Pericardial effusion common, tamponade rare; syst/diastolic dysfunction; $\uparrow$ cholesterol → accelerated atherosclerosis & risk of MI • **GI:** obstipation/constipation • **Renal:** hyponatremia with $\uparrow$ total body Na – accumulated in myxedema • **Exam:** Dry, coarse, scaly skin; surgical scar on neck; pseudomyotonia; sparse or coarse hair, carotinemic pallor, puffy facies, enlarged tongue, hoarseness, moderate-profound hypotension without shivering • **Labs:** $\downarrow$ Glc; $\downarrow$ Na; $\uparrow$ K; $\uparrow$ cortisol; $\uparrow$ Hct; $\uparrow$ WBC; Cr > 2; $\uparrow$ P_aCO_2; $\downarrow$ P_aO_2

Management
- Replace thyroid hormone. **Thyroxine** (T4) has $t_{1/2} \sim 7d$, must be converted to T3 for activity. Load 4 μg/kg or 500 μg IV or po then 50-100 μg qd. **Triiodothyronine** (T3): active hormone, $t_{1/2} \sim 1d$. Danger of rapid $\uparrow$ metabolic demand and acute myocardial ischemia. Generally avoided except in life-threatening hypothyroidism in which (1) slow-onset of T4 monotherapy poses unacceptable delay, or (2) concurrent severe nonthyroidal illness inhibits peripheral T4→T3 conversion, rendering T4 administration futile. Dose 25 μg po/IV q 6h until response.
- Concurrent adrenal insufficiency common (5-10%) → initial **IV glucocorticoids**
- Expedite mechanical ventilation for respiratory failure: rapid progression; aspiration risk high; occ upper airway obstruction; $\downarrow$ surfactant produced
- Hemodynamic collapse: consider pericardiocentesis; usually already vasoconstricted, use volume >> α-adrenergic agents
- Hypothermia: use blankets; risk distributive shock from external warming
- Volume overload is uncommon; diuretics risk further $\downarrow$ cardiac output
- Hyponatremia: treat with free-water restriction; total body Na-overloaded
- Search for precipitant and consider empiric antimicrobial therapy
- Drug metabolism is reduced; care in choosing proper dose of all drugs
- Prophylax against gastritis & ulcers • Correct anemia
- Note dopamine inhibits TSH production
- Consider baseline cardiac isoenzymes before thyroid replacement

[89] L Wartowsky, "Myxedema coma," in *Werner and Ingbar's Thyroid: a fundamental and clinical text*, 6/e, LE Braverman & RD Utiger (eds), Philadelphia : Lippincott, 1991. RE Weiss and S Refeluff, "Hypothyroidism, nonthyroidal illness, and myxedema coma," in *Principles of critical care*, JB Hill, GA Schmidt, L Wood (eds), NY:McGraw-Hill, 1992. MacKerrow SD, *et al*, "Myxedema-associated cardiogenic shock treated with intravenous triiodothyronine," *Ann Intern Med*, 1992;117(12):1014-5.

Thyroid Storm[90]

Precipitants: Infection; surgery; trauma; iodinated contrast dye; hypoglycemia; parturition; vigorous thyroid palpation; psychiatric stress; withdrawal of antithyroid drugs; ^{131}I-therapy; DKA; PE; stroke; health-food containing seaweed or kelp

Features
- Fever, tachycardia, diaphoresis out of proportion to apparent infection, often metabolic-pattern encephalopathy, hypertension, $\downarrow SaO_2$
- Suggestive of dx: Previous thyrotoxicosis; Exophthalmos or goiter; Use of thyroid hormone; Surgical neck scar; Recent iodine-radiocontrast agents
- Cardiopulmonary: $\uparrow$ metabolic demand, $\uparrow O_2$ consumption; $\uparrow$ cardiac output; Hyperdynamic circulation and high-output CHF; Myocardial ischemia; Arrhythmias (usually supraventricular); $\uparrow$ work of breathing & respiratory muscle weakness;
- Neurologic: Myopathy > 50%; Exophthalmic ophthalmoplegia; Aggravated myasthenia gravis; Thyrotoxic periodic paralysis (Asian men); Sensorium: delirium, stupor, coma, seizures
- GI: Hypermotility with malabsorption; Hypergastrinemia → PUD
- Labs: $\uparrow$ T4, $\uparrow$ FT4I, $\uparrow$ T3, $\uparrow$ Glc, $\uparrow$ WBC with shift, anemia, $\downarrow$ platelets, $\downarrow$ K, $\uparrow$ Ca (may be severe) , abnormal liver enzymes, $\uparrow$ cortisol

Antithyroid measures
- Block production of thyroid hormone:
  - Propylthiouracil po/NG/pr 200-250 mg q 4h. Inhibits T4→T3 conversion. Does not affect release of preformed T4 stores.
  - Methimazole 20-25mg po (40mg crushed in NS pr q6h). Does not inhibit T4→T3 conversion. Does not affect release of preformed T4.
- Block release of T3 & T4 by thyroid into blood
  - SSKI 8 drops q 6h or NaI 0.5-1.0 g IV q 12. **Caution:** Use only after methimazole or PTU. **Not** for monotherapy, can exacerbate thyrotoxicosis.
- Lithium carbonate if allergic to I: 300 mg q 6h to keep level ~ 1mEq/L

Other management issues
- β-adrenergic blockers to $\downarrow$ cardiovascular effects (eg propranolol, esmolol) until bradycardic. If bronchospasm, consider reserpine (1 mg IM test then 2.5-5 mg IM q 4h). For CHF, use inotropes >> afterload agents.
- Control hyperthermia with acetaminophen not salicylates. Control shivering with IV meperidine and chlorpromazine (? report of dantrolene)
- Fluid resuscitation + dextrose for diaphoresis, vomiting, diarrhea, hypoglycemia
- Parenteral vitamin supplements (eg B-complex)
- Glucocorticoids empirically for relative adrenal insufficiency & to $\downarrow$ T4 → T3

Adrenal Crisis[91]

Setting
- Sudden extensive adrenal destruction or chronic/established <u>primary</u> adrenal insufficiency after major physiologic stress (eg surgery, infection) without adequate glucocorticoid replacement.

---

[90] L Wartowsky, "Thyrotoxic storm," in <u>Werner and Ingbar's Thyroid: a fundamental and clinical text</u>, 6/e, LE Braverman & RD Utiger (eds), Philadelphia : Lippincott, 1991. RE Weiss and S Refeluff, "Thyrotoxicosis," in <u>Principles of critical care</u>, JB Hill, GA Schmidt, L Wood (eds), NY:McGraw-Hill, 1992.
[91] Orth DN, et al, "The adrenal cortex," in Wilson JD, Foster DW, (eds.), <u>Williams textbook of endocrinology</u>, 8/e., Philadelphia: Saunders, 1992. Burke CW, "Adrenocortical insufficiency," <u>Clin Endocrinol Metab</u>, 1985; 14(4):947-976. Aron DC, "Metabolic and endocrine emergencies," in Saunders CE, Ho MT (eds.), <u>Current Emergency Diagnosis and Treatment</u>, 4/e, Norwalk, CT: Appleton & Lange, 1992.

- Uncommon in secondary/tertiary adrenal insufficiency because of preserved renin-angiotensin-aldosterone axis. However, previous glucocorticoid tx can suppress pituitary-adrenal axis, even after short treatment, low doses[92].
- Mineralocorticoid → intravascular volume; Glucocorticoid → vascular tone.

Etiology

- Bilateral adrenal infarction: • Hemorrhagic (anticoagulation, coagulopathy, perioperative) often occult, • Thrombotic (adrenal vein thrombosis after back injury); • Sepsis: meningococcemia (Waterhouse-Friederichsen), Pseudomonas.
- Autoimmune adrenalitis • Autoimmune polyglandular failure • Granulomatous infection, eg tuberculosis, histoplasmosis & other fungi • HIV • Drug inhibition of cortisol synthesis (Ketoconazole, etomidate, aminoglutethimide, metyrapone) • Drug acceleration of cortisol degredation in setting of mild adrenal insufficiency (phenytoin, rifampin, barbiturates). • Pituitary apoplexy

Symptoms and signs

- Dehydration & hypotension out of proportion to severity of acute illness, seemingly unresponsive to fluids; Shock is not always heralded by symptomatic hypotension. • Nausea & vomiting with history of anorexia and weight loss • Unexplained fever • Severe abdominal pain & nonlocalizing tenderness, may mimic surgical emergency. • Hyponatremia (compensatory ↑ ADH), hyperkalemia (↓ aldosterone), azotemia, eosinophilia, hypoglycemia, hypercalcemia • Hyperpigmentation mucosae, creases, & sun-spared skin (in 1° disease). • Concurrent hypothyroidism or hypogonadism in polyendocrine syndromes • Altered sensorium • Small cardiac silhouette on CXR • Calcified adrenals (in infection), Adrenal mass on CT (in hemorrhage, tumor)
- Secondary adrenal insufficiency differs in that • Pro-opiomelanocortinin not elevated • Hyperkalemia does not occur & Azotemia uncommon with preserved mineralocorticoid activity • Hyponatremia from ↑ ADH • Hypoglycemia common

Diagnosis • Random "Stressed" Cortisol level < 5 µg/dL: During stress "If [cortisol] ain't high, it's low.[93]" • Cortrosyn (synthetic ACTH) stimulation: 1 mg SQ/IM/IV should double serum cortisol to ≥ 20 µg/dL after 60 min • Prolonged ACTH infusion may be necessary to distinguish 1° from 2° or 3° disease.

Therapy: (1) Restore vascular volume and tone before diagnosis (2) Diagnosis (3) Replace mineralocorticoid (4) Treat precipitant.

- RAPID volume resuscitation to restore 50% circulating volume (typically 2-3 L NS) titrated to JVP or pulmonary edema. Replace K, glucose prn.
- Vasopressors don't work well without glucocorticoid replacement.
- Dexamethasone (5 mg IV) will not interfere with serum cortisol measurements but has no mineralocorticoid activity. Use Hydrocortisone 100 mg IV q 6-8h after ACTH stim tests. Avoid cortisone (prodrug requires hepatic metabolism).
- Serum K may be elevated, but total body K often depleted by GI illness.
- Mineralocorticoid after volume resuscitation: fludrocortisone (Florinef) ~0.1 mg/d.
- Identify and treat precipitating illness.

---

92 Schlaghecke R, et al, "The effect of long-term glucocorticoid therapy on pituitary-adrenal responses to exogenous corticotropin-releasing hormone," N Engl J Med, 1992;326(4):226-30.
93 DC Aron, Case Western Reserve University School of Medicine, typical sage advice.

Pituitary Apoplexy[94]

Setting · Hemorrhagic infarction of (usually tumor-laden) pituitary.
· Precipitated by anticoagulation (including CABG surgery), irradiation, Sheehan syndrome (peripartum vasospastic pituitary infarction usually with hypotension), hormone therapy (estrogen, prostate suppression), surgery (as with Sheehan syndrome), trauma

Manifestations
· Intracerebral hemorrhage: Meningeal irritation, headache, CSF xanthochromia
· Expanding intrasellar mass: Headache, diplopia, bitemporal visual field deficits, extraocular muscle palsy, altered sensorium or coma, central respiratory failure, hyponatremia (SIADH)
· Acute panhypopituitarism: Hypotension (adrenal), hypernatremia (DI)

Treatment · Hemodynamic resuscitation with volume, electrolyte therapy
· Glucocorticoid replacement (hydrocortisone 100 mg IV q 6-8h)
· Accurate diagnostic studies (CT, MRI)

Gastroenterology

Pancreatitis: Prognosis

Ranson Criteria predictive of poor prognosis[95]
· Upon arrival: (1) Age > 55 yrs; (2) WBC > 16,000; (3) Blood glucose > 200 mg/dL; (4) Serum LDH > twice normal; (5) Serum AST > six times normal; (5) Other non-Ranson indicators of poor prognosis: hypotension, pulmonary disease, palpable abdominal mass, hemorrhagic ascites, first attack
· First 48 hours: (1) Hematocrit < 30% or fall > 10%; (2) Serum calcium < 8 mg/dL; (3) BUN increase > 5 mg/dL; (4) Arterial pO_2 < 60 mm Hg; (5) Base deficit > 4 mEq/l; (6) Estimated fluid sequestration > 6 liters; (7) Massive volume resuscitation
· Prognosis[96]

Risk factors	Mortality	% Dead or > 7d in ICU
0-2	3 (0.9%)	13 (3.7%)
3-4	11 (16%)	27 (40%)
5-6	12 (40%)	28 (93%)
7-8	6 (100%)	6 (100%)

94 Reid RL, et al, "Pituitary apoplexy. A review," Arch Neurol, 1985;42(7):712-9. Aron DC, "Metabolic and endocrine emergencies," in Saunders CE, Ho MT (eds.), Current Emergency Diagnosis and Treatment, 4/e, Norwalk, CT: Appleton & Lange, 1992. Vidal E, et al, "Twelve cases of pituitary apoplexy," Arch Intern Med, 1992;152(9):1893-9. Maccagnan P, et al, "Conservative management of pituitary apoplexy," J Clin Endocrinol Metab, 1995;80(7):2190-7.
95 JHC Ranson, et al, Surg Gynecol Obstet 143:209, 1976.
96 JHC Ranson, FC Spencer, Ann Surg 187:565, 1978.

Surgical Risk in Liver Disease[97]

Child-Turcotte Classification[98]

	Class A	Class B	Class C
Bilirubin (mg/dL)	<2.0	2.0-3.0	>3.0
Albumin (g/dL)	>3.5	3.0-3.5	<3.0
Ascites	None	Easily controlled	Poorly controlled
Encephalopathy	None	Mild	Advanced
Nutrition	Excellent	Good	Poor

Pugh's classification[99]

	1 point	2 pts	3 pts	
Encephalopathy	None	1-2	3-4	**Class A:**5-6 pts
Ascites	Absent	Slight	Moderate	**Class B:**7-9 pts
Bilirubin (mg/dL for PBC)	1-2	2-3	>3	**Class C:**10-15
Albumin (g/dL)	3.5	2.8-3.5	<2.8	
PT prolongation (s)	1-4	4-6	>6	

Encephalopathy

I: Prodrome. Euphoria, occ depression; fluctuant mild confusion; slowed mentation & affect; slurred speech; disordered sleep rhythm; sl asterixis.
II: Impending coma. Drowsy; inappropriate behav; incontinent. Asterixis.
III: Highly somnolent but arousable; incoherent speech; marked confusion.
IV: A:Responds B:Unresponsive to painful stimuli.

Operability[100]

Class A: Normal response to all operations, normal regenerative ability.
Class B: Mod liver impairment. Tolerates surgery only with preop preparation. Limited regeneration; sizable resections contraindicated.
Class C: Poor response to all operations regardless of preparatory efforts, liver resection regardless of size is contraindicated.

Peritonitis in cirrhotic with ascites[101]

	SBP	Surgical peritonitis
Pneumoperitoneum	Never	Usual
Polymicrobial infection	Rare	Common
Candida in ascites	Rare	Occasional
Ascitic protein	< 1g/dl	>1g/dl
Ascitic glucose	>50mg/dl	<50mg/dl
Fever, pain, ileus	NSD	NSD

---

[97] Friedman LS, Maddrey WC, "Surgery in the patient with liver disease," Med Clin North Am, 1987;71(3):453.
[98] Child G & Turcotte, "Surgery and portal hypertension," in Child The Liver and Portal Hypertension, Philadelphia: Saunders, 1964.
[99] Pugh, "Transection of the oesophagus for bleeding oesophageal varices," Br J Surg (NY: Churchill-Livingstone) 1973;60:646.
[100] Stone, "Preoperative and postoperative care," Surg Clin North Am, 1977;57:409.
[101] Gholson et al, "Hepatological considerations in patients with parenchymal liver disease undergoing surgery," Am J Gastroenterology, 85:487, 1990.

Nutrition Calculations[102]

Total Caloric Requirements
- Simple estimation for ICU patients:
  - <u>Calories</u>: 20-25 (mild stress), 25-35 (typical ICU pt), 40-50 (severe stress) kcal/kg/day.   Rarely > 1700 kcal or 100 g protein/d
  - <u>Protein</u> 1.25-1.5g/kg; uremia not dialyzed: 0.8g/kg; dialysis:1.0-1.5 g/kg
  - <u>Fluid</u> typically 30 ml/kg/d
- **OR** Harris-Benedict basal energy requirements kcal/d
  - Men: 13.8×Weight (kg) + 5×Height (cm) - 6.76×Age (yrs) + 66.5
  - Women: 9.56×Weight (kg) + 1.86×Height (cm) - 4.68×Age (yrs) + 655
  - **Stress factor:**[103]

Mild starvation	0.85-1.10	Severe infection	1.30-1.55
Postop uncomplicated	1.0-1.05	Cancer	1.1-1.45
Peritonitis	1.05-1.25	Burn/severe trauma	? 1.75

Parenteral nutrition components
- Glucose: Anhydrous 4 kcal/g; Hydrated 3.4 kcal/g
  - Infuse 4-5 mg/kg/min, "optimum" minimizing hepatic steatosis risk
- Triglycerides (Long-chain): 9 kcal/g as lipid emulsion, usual minimum 10% caloric intake, max 2.5g/kg/d or up to 60% of daily caloric intake
- IV Amino acids: 4 kcal/g, typically 40-50 g/L.

Common parenteral solutions

Dextrose	Kcal/L	mOsm/L
5%	170	250
10%	340	500

Lipid	Kcal/L	mOsm/L
10%	1100	280
20%	2000	330-340

TPN solutions	Protein	Dextrose	Kcal/L
Central formula II	50 g/L	25%	1050
Central formula I	42.5 g/L	25%	1020
Peripheral	42.5 g/L	10%	510

Start TPN @ ~50cc/h, ↑ ~25 cc/hr qd. Infuse lipids over 10-24h qd/qod.

Enteral Feeding Commercial Products

	Kcal/mL	Protein (g/L)	mOsm/L
Jevity/Osmolite/Osmolite HN	1.06	37-44	300-310
Pulmocare (Low resp quotient)	1.5	63	490
Magnacal	2.0	70	590
Vital (Elemental)	1.0	42	500

Begin half/full-strength @ 50cc/hr, ↑ by 25cc/hr q 12 hr. √ Residuals q 4 hr, hold feeding 1 hr for residual > 100cc then resume. Elevate HOB>30º.

Nitrogen Balance = (Protein intake (grams) / 6.25 - (UUN + 4)
- 6.25 reflects that Protein ≈ 16% N; 4 reflect obligatory N loss in skin/stool
- Goal = 0; Moderate stress 0-5; Severe stress > 5

---

[102] RE Clouse, "Nutrional therapy," in WC Dunagan *et al*, (eds) <u>Manual of Medical Therapeutics</u>, Boston: Little, Brown, 1989. Cindy Hamilton, "Nutritional support for the critically ill patient," 1991, Univ Hospitals Cleveland.

[103] James L Rippe, *et al* "Intensive Care Medicine," 2/e, p1670, Boston:Little-Brown, 1991.

Hematology-Oncology

Hemolytic Anemia[104]

Mechanistic classification
- **Extrinsic**
  - Splenomegaly
  - Antibody-mediated
    - **Warm**-antibody immunohemolytic anemia: Idiopathic; Lymphomas (CLL, NHL, advanced Hodgkin infrequent); SLE; Tumors (rare)
      Drugs: **(1)** Methyldopa-type: resembles idiopathic (above); **(2)** Penicillin type: hapten-mediated; **(3)** "Bystander"-type (uncommon, seen with drugs: quinin/idine, INH, sulfonamides, p-ASA, insecticides): IgG or IgM, capable of complement fixation. antibody-antigen complex dissociates leaving only C3
    - **Cold**-antibody immunohemolytic anemia
      - Cold agglutinin disease: • Acute: mycoplasma infection, infectious mononucleosis • Chronic: Idiopathic, lymphoma
      - Paroxysmal cold hemoglobinuria: Donath-Landsteiner IgG in tertiary syphilis, acute viral syndromes (*eg* measles, mumps)
  - Mechanical trauma: microangiopathic hemolytic anemia
    - March hemoglobinuria • Cardiac valvular stenosis or prosthesis
    - Endothelial dz: malignant HTN, eclampsia, renal graft rejection, hemangioma, scleroderma, TTP / HUS, DIC
  - Toxin-effect: malaria, clostridial infection, bacteremia, brown-recluse spider, copper toxicity including Wilson's disease, extensive burns
- **Membrane abnormalities**: Paroxysmal nocturnal hemoglobinuria; Hereditary spherocytosis, elliptocytosis, stomatocytosis; Spur cell anemia
- **Hereditary RBC defects**: Hemoglobinopathy; G-6-PD deficiency; PK deficiency

G-6-PD deficiency and drugs[105]
- Drugs associated with **hemolysis** in G-6-PD deficiency: Doxorubicin; methylene blue; nalidixic acid; nitrofurantoin; primaquine; sulfamethoxazole; Fava beans (though most pts are not susceptible; other host factors probably involved)
- Drugs **safe** in G-6-PD deficiency (past warnings attributable to infective hemolysis): acetaminophen; ascorbate; aspirin; chloramphenicol; chloroquine; colchicine; diphenhydramine; isoniazid; phenytoin; probencid; procainamide; pyrimethamine; quinine/dine; streptomycin; sulfisoxazole; trimethoprim; vitamin K

Iron-Deficiency Anemia

Absorption & Transport:
- Duodenum/upper jejunum. Ferric (Fe^{3+}) most common in diet, solubilized by gastric acid. Of 10-20mg/d ingested, 10-20% absorbed.
- Absorption ↑ by citrate & ascorbate, ↓ by tannate (tea), plant phytates, PO_4.
- Transferrin binds Fe once translocated across gut epithelium.
- Excess iron stored as **Ferritin**: levels reflect total body iron stores; **Hemosiderin**: "dump" form not easily metabolically accessible

---

[104] RA Cooper, HF Bunn, "Hemolytic anemias," in JD Wilson *et al* (eds), Harrison's Principles of Internal Medicine 12th 1991,NY:McGraw-Hill.
[105] E Beutler, "Glucose-6-Phosphate dehydrogenase deficiency," N Engl J Med 324(3):170-4, 1991.

Assays of iron stores
- **Direct: Liver biopsy.** Prussian blue stain of nonformalin specimens, only semiquantitative. Best: atomic absorption spectroscopy of formalin specimens. **Bone marrow** good in Fe-deficiency, unreliable in Fe-excess.
- **Indirect: Serum Transferrin & Iron:** Fe saturation < 10%, transferrin elevated in Fe-deficiency; **Circulatory ferritin:** increased with Fe-loading, but acute-phase reactant. **Protoporphyrin IX (FEP),** accumulates in RBCs in Fe-deficiency, cheap screen. **CT liver** (dual energy): good assessment of iron-overload.

Etiologies
- Increased utilitization: Postnatal or adolescent growth spurt
- Physiologic loss: Menstruation; Pregnancy
- Decreased intake: **Malabsorption:** Primary malabsorption; S/p gastrectomy, causes shortened transit time; S/p duodenal/jejunal resection; Achlorhydria: dietary Ferric needs acidification. Note Fe-deficiency → achlorhydria. **Meat-poor diets**
- Pathologic loss: **GI:** Hookworm; CA; PUD/gastritis/AVM; Rare: NSAID, hemorrhoid; **GU** (not occult); **Lung** (hemosiderosis, bronchiectasis)

Manifestations
- GI (high epithelial turnover): Glossitis (tender, shiny, smooth tongue with papillary erosions), angular chelitis, gastric atrophy with secondary achlorhydria, postcricoid anterior web (Plummer-Vinson). • Menorrhagia • Koilonychia (slowing of nail plate growth) • Pica: starch, ice, clay; may cause lead ingestion

Natural history
(1) Storage depletion (decreased marrow stores and ferritin levels)
(2) Abnormal erythropoiesis: Increased TIBC, decreased iron, increased FEP, then microcytosis & hypochromia. (3) Anemia

Iron supplementation
- Reticulocytosis 3-4d, max 10d
- Failure to respond: wrong diagnosis, noncompliance, loss exceeds replacement, bone marrow is suppressed, malabsorption

Sideroblastic anemia

Description
- Defective Fe utilization with impaired hemoglobin synthesis and accumulation of surplus iron with arrested maturation of erythroblasts. Causes spurious appearance of erythroid hyperplasia on Bx. Marrow erythroblasts show arc of $FePO_4$ deposits within mitochondria in ring around nucleus.
- Characteristics: hypochromic, microcytic RBC's with increased serum ferritin and increased tissue iron stores.
- Idiosyncratic response (~5%) to pyridoxine therapy, not reflective of pyridoxine deficiency.

Differential diagnosis
- Congenital
- Acquired
) Toxic: •EtOH: resolves after cessation •Lead: Neuropathy, abdominal colic, gout, hypochromic anemia •Isoniazid & anti-tuberculous drugs (uncommon) •Chloramphenicol
) Inflammatory: cancer, collagen vascular) Idiopathic
) Alkylating agent: refractory to B6, progresses to AML within months.

Therapy
- Withdraw offending agent   ) Trial of 3 months 100-200mg daily pyridoxine.
- Consider concommitant folate replacement   ) If idiopathic and transfusion-dependent, consider androgens and consider deferoxamine.

Megaloblastic anemias[106]

Etiologies
<u>Vitamin B12 deficiency</u> (Serum < 100 pMol; < 150 pg/ml)
- Inadequate diet or increased requirements
- Deficiency of gastric intrinsic factor: gastrectomy, pernicious anemia
- Malabsorption: ileitis/resection, diphyllobothrum latum, bactovergrowth

<u>Folate deficiency</u> (Serum < 3 ng/mL)
- Consumption: pregnancy, hemolytic anemia, hyper/myeloproliferative
- Malabsorption: Sprue, extensive small bowel disease/resection/fistulae, anticonvulsants, oral contraceptives

<u>Drug-induced suppression of DNA synthesis</u>
- Folate antagonists: trimethoprim, methotrexate, pyrimethamine, EtOH
- Metabolic inhibitors: of purine, pyrimidine, thymidylate synthesis: 6-MP, azathioprine, 5-FU, hydroxyurea, ara-C, AZT; Alkylating agents
- Nitrous oxide (rapidly inhibits methionine synthetase)

<u>Congenital</u>: Lesch-Nyhan; Oritic aciduria; Folate metabolism; B12 transport
<u>Erythroleukemia</u> (M6 AML)
<u>Spurious</u>: Antibiotics reduce folate microbiological assay;

Diagnosis
- Chemistries: LDH ↑ ~fifteen-fold; ↑ Ferritin saturation; ↓ haptoglobin
- Peripheral smear evidence of megaloblastic "arrest:" hypersegmented neutrophils & macroovalocytes (egg shaped, not elliptocytes)
- Marrow: Imbalance of nuclear/cellular maturation, obvious in most mature cells. Hypercellular, erythroid marrow.   Intramedullary hemolysis of ineffective erythropoiesis. Giant band forms and metamyelocytes.
- Schilling test: **(1)** 1-2µg radiocobalt-labelled B12 *po* + supraphysiologic *IM* B12 to saturate B12 binding sites. Low 24-48 hr urinary excretion (<7%) suggests malabsoprtion. Verify collection: 24hr urine creatinine.
  (2) Repeat 5 days later, with purified intrinsic factor (60 mg) po. Normalization of urinary excretion diagnoses pernicious anemia
  (3) Repeat tetracycline 250 mg qid x 10d: normalization ← bacterial overgrowth
- Therepeutic trial: Reticulocytosis ← 0.2-0.4µg (low/physiologic) folate or 1-2µg B12 IM. Inaccurate w/o rigorous diet/blood observation 1-2 wks.

Neuropsychiatric manifestations of B12 deficiency
- <u>Myelopathy</u>: <u>Posterior columns</u>: acroparesthesias fingers & toes; incoordination legs>arms; ↓ position & vibration sense; sensory ataxia leg>arms. <u>Lateral columns</u>: Generalized weakness legs > arms. <u>Spinothalamic</u>: nocturnal cramps, tabetic-type abdominal crises
- <u>Encephalopathy</u>: Dementia; Personality Δ (apathy, irritability, lability); Cranial neuropathy: altered taste & smell
- <u>Peripheral neuropathy</u> (may be related to myelopathy): acroparesthesias legs > arms; dimished vibration & proprioception legs first; ↓ DTRs

---

[106] James H. Jandl, <u>Blood: Textbook of Hematology</u>, Boston: Little, Brown & Co, 1987.

Leukemia, Acute Myelogenous[107]

Classification

No Periodic-Acid-Schiff-staining or common ALL Antigen (CALLA) or terminal deoxynucleotidase or immunoglobulin-gene rearrangement seen in AML
AML (not megakaryoblastic) stains myeloperoxidase (MPO) & myeloerythroid (ME) markers

FAB morphology	MPO/ME stain	Surface Antigens	Clinical syndromes
M0 Undifferentiated	-/-	CD13, CD33	
M1 Myeloid without maturation	+/-	CD13, CD33	
M2 Myeloid with maturation	+/-	CD13, CD33	
M3 Acute promyelocytic	+/-	CD13, CD33, CD15	DIC common
M4 Myelomonocytic; M4 Eosinophil variant(25%)	+/+	Granulocytic & Monocytic markers	M4Eo marrow eosinophilia & CNS myeloblastomas
M5 Monocytic	+/+	Monocytic markers CD11b, My8, CD14	Gum/skin infiltrates; increased lysozyme
M6 Erythroleukemia	+/-	Glycophorin	Evolves from CML & myelodysplasia; transforms to M1,2
M7 Megakaryoblastic	-/-	Factors 7 & 8 Ag, CD42	Myelofibrosis (dry taps) common

Therapy • Control blast crisis (>100k) with hydroxyurea & leukapheresis
  • Intensive induction (usually ara-C & anthracycline) -> complete remission 60-80%
  • Consolidation/intensification to eradicate ~ 10^7 cells; LTS ?15-20%
  • Adverse prognosticators: age > 45; hx treatment-induced myelodysplasia
  • Median duration complete remission ~1-2 yrs   • Autologous marrow transplant
  • Allogeneic marrow transplant: efficacy depends on graft-vs-leukemia
   • 1/3 adults<45 die peritransplant; therefore only age < 45   • GVHD
   • marrow transplant accessible for only 10% AML
  • Differentiating agents, eg trans-retinoic acid induces differentiation of M3

Staging Lymphoma[108]

Rye Classification of Hodgkin Disease

Histologic group	%	R-S cells	Other pathology	Prognosis
Lymphocyte-predominant	2-10	Rare	Mostly normal-appearing lymphocytes	Excellent
Nodular sclerosis	40-80	Frequent "lacunae"	Lymphoid nodules, collagen bands	Very good
Mixed cellularity	20-40	Numerous	Pleomorphic infiltrate	Good
Lymphocyte-depleted	2-15	Numerous, often bizarre	Paucity of lymphocytes, pleomorphic, fibrosis	Poor

---

[107] Mastrianni DM, Tung NM, Tenen DG, "Acute myelogenous leukemia: current treatment and future directions," Am J Med, 92(3):286-95, 1992.
[108] LM Nadler, "The malignant lymphomas," in JD Wilson et al (eds), Harrison's Principles of Internal Medicine 12/e 1991,NY:McGraw-Hill.

Histological classification of non-Hodgkin lymphoma

Working formulation	Rappaport terminology	5-yr survival
Low-grade		
Small lymphocytic cell	Diffuse well-diff'd lymphocytic	60%
Follicular, predominantly small cleaved cell	Nodular poorly differentiated lymphocytic	70%
Follicular mixed, small cleaved & large cell	Nodular mixed lymphocytic histiocytic	50%
Intermediate grade		
Follicular, predominantly. large cell	Nodular histiocytic	44%
Diffuse small cleaved cell	Diffuse poorly differentiated lymphocytic	35%
Diffuse mixed, small & large cell	Diffuse mixed lympho- & histiocytic	40%
Diffuse large cell	Diffuse histiocytic	34%
High-grade		
Large cell immunoblastic	Diffuse histiocytic	30%
Lymphoblastic	Diffuse lymphoblastic	24%
Small noncleaved cell; Burkitt's	Diffuse undifferentiated	23%

Ann Arbor Staging for Hodgkin and non-Hodgkin Lymphoma

Stage I	Single lymph node region or single extralymphatic site
Stage II	Two or more LN regions on the same side of the diaphragm. Can also include localized extralymphatic site (Stage IIE).
Stage III	LN regions or extralymphatic sites on both sides of diaphragm.
Stage IV	One or more extralymphatic organs with or without LN involvement.

Substage **A**: Asymptomatic; **B**: Hx of fever, sweats, weight loss > 10% body weight

Staging Lung Cancer[109]

Tx	Malignant cells found but not visualized radiographically or bronchoscopically
T0	No evidence of primary tumor
Tis	Carcinoma in situ
T1	Tumor < 3.0cm surrounded by lung or visceral pleura, without evidence of invasion proximal to a lobar bronchus at bronchoscopy.
T2	Tumor > 3.0 cm, or either invades visceral pleura or has associated atelectasis or obstructive pneumonitis extending to the hilar region. At bronchoscopy, proximal extent must be within a lobar bronchus or at least 2.0 cm beyond carina. Any associated atelectasis or obstructive pneumonitis must involve less than an entire lung.
T3	Tumor of any size with direct extension into the chest wall (including superior sulcus tumors), diaphragm, mediastinal pleura or pericardium without involving the heart, great vessels, trachea, esophagus or vertebral body, or a tumor in the main bronchus within 2 cm of the carina without involving the carina.
T4	Worse than T3, or invasion or carina, or malignant pleural effusion.
N0	No demonstrable metastases to regional nodes.
N1	Mets to peribronchial and/or ipsilateral hilar LNs, including direct extension.
N2	Mets to ipsilateral mediastinal & subcarinal LN's
N3	Mets to contralateral mediastinal, contralateral hilar, ipsilateral or contralateral scalene or supraclavicular LNs.
M0	No (known) distant metastases
M1	Distant metastasis present

[109] HJ Tabbarah, BB Lowitz, DA Casciato, "Lung cancer," in DA Casciato & BA Lowitz, <u>Manual of Clinical Oncology</u>, 2/e, Boston: Little, Brown, 1988.

Prognosis & Survival by Stage

Stage I	T1N0M0	80-90% (5 yr)	
	T2N0M0	40-50% (5 yr)	
Stage II	T1N1M0	30-40% (5 yr)	Resectable
	T2N1M0	20% (5 yr)	
Stage IIIa	T3N0M0, T3N1M0, T1-3N2M0	8-10% (5 yr)	
Stage IIIb	TanyN3M0, T4NanyM0	9-12 mo (median)	Unresectable
Stage IV	TanyNanyM1	6-9 mo (median)	

Median survival of untreated lung cancer pts

Karnofsky scale	Confined to one hemithorax	Extensive disease
10-40	10 wks	2 wks
50-70	20 wks	10 wks
80-100	30 wks	20 wks

Unresectability: • Small cell CA • Distant mets including opposite lung • Pleural effusion ± malignant cells • Supraclavicular or contralateral mediastinal LN involvement (bx proven) • Recurrent laryngeal nerve • Tracheal wall • ? Mainstem bronchus < 2cm from carina

Staging Renal Cancer[110]

Stage	Extent	5-yr survival	10-yr survival
I	Confined to renal parenchyma	65-70%	55-60%
II	Into perirenal fat but confined to Gerota's fascia	50%	20%
III	Extends into renal vein or IVC	50%	35%
	Involves LNs or other vascular structures	35%	-
IV	Invades adjacent organs or has distant metastases	<10%	-

Prognosis
• Without treatment, survival <5% at 3 yrs; <2% at 5 yrs (without staging)
• Histology: clear-cell best; undiff'd & spindle-cell 5-yr survival < 25%
• Venous extension: not hopeless

Staging Colon Cancer[111]

TNM Definitions

TX	Primary tumor cannot be assessed	NX	Regional nodes cannot be assessed	MX	Cannot be assessed
T0	No evidence of primary tumor	N0	No node metastasis	M0	No distant metastasis
Tis	Carcinoma *in situ* not extending through muscularis	N1	1-3 pericolic or perirectal lymph nodes	M1	Distant metastasis
T1	Invades submucosa	N2	>3 pericolic or perirectal lymph nodes		
T2	Invades muscularis	N3	Along named vascular trunk or apical node		
T3	Into subserosa or nonperitonealized pericolic or perirectal tissue				
T3	Into other structures or visceral perforation				

[110] JB deKernion, BB Lowitz, DA Casciato, "Urinary tract cancers," in DA Casciato & BA Lowitz, Manual of Clinical Oncology, 2/e, Boston: Little, Brown, 1988.
[111] American Joint Committee on Cancer, Beahrs OH (ed), Manual for staging of cancer, Philadelphia: JB Lippincott, 1992; BB Lowitz & DA Casciato, "Gastrointestinal tract cancers," in DA Casciato & BA Lowitz, Manual of Clinical Oncology, 2/e, Boston: Little, Brown, 1988.

Stage Grouping

AJCC/UICC	T	N	M	Dukes
Stage 0	Tis	N0	M0	—
Stage I	T1, T2	N0	M0	A
Stage II	T3, T4	N0	M0	B
Stage III	Tany	N1, N2, N3	M0	C
Stage IV	Tany	Nany	M1	D

Survival by Stage in 111,110 patients 1973-87

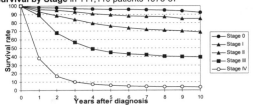

Other prognostic factors

- Histologic grade · Well-differentiated (G1, G2): 5-yr survival 55%
  · Poorly-differentiated (G3, G4): 5-yr survival 30%
- High CEA (>10ng/ml) preop: higher risk of relapse
- Invasive tumors worse than tumors that push surrrounding tissue
- Venous invasion associated with high risk of metastases
- Selected syndromes & median survival · GI symptoms, stage C disease or direct extension to surrounding organs: 10-12 mo · Liver involvement or peritoneal seeding: 7-8 mo · Ascites or extraabdominal mets: 4-5 mo

Staging Prostate Cancer[112]

Stage	Extent / Proportion of pts	10-yr survival	
A	Incidental histological finding; nl palpation (10%)	60%	
A1	Single focal area of well-differentiated tumor		
A2	Multiple foci or poorly-differentiated tumor		
B	Tumor palpable but confined to prostate (10%)	40%	
B1	Single nodule < 2 cm diameter		
B2	Multiple nodules or single nodule > 2 cm		
C	Localized to periprostatic area (45%)	30%	
C1	Seminal vesicles not involved & tumor < 70g		
C2	Seminal vesicles involved & tumor < 70 g		
D	Advanced disease (35%)	10-20%	Inoperable
D1	Pelvic node metastases or ureteral obstruction		
D2	Distant metastases		

---

[112] JB deKernion, et al, "Urinary tract cancers," in DA Casciato & BA Lowitz, Manual of Clinical Oncology 2/e., Boston: Little, Brown, 1988.

Staging Ovarian Cancer[113]

FIGO Stage	Extent	%	5-yr survival
I	Ovaries only	15	80%
a	1 ovary, no ascites or tumor on ext. surface, ext. capsule intact		
b	2 ovaries, no ext. surface ascites or tumor, ext. capsule intact		
c	Ia or Ib + surface tumor on 1 or 2 ovaries or capsule ruptured or with malignant cells in ascites or peritoneal washings		
II	Extension into true pelvis	10	60%
a	Extension/metastasis to uterus and/or tubes		
b	Extension to other pelvic tissues		
c	(IIa or IIb) and Ic		
III	Extension or metastasis into abd. cavity including metastatic implantation on peritoneal surfaces of liver, diaphragm, & serosal surface of bowel	70	40%
a	Macroscopically limited to true pelvis with (-) nodes and with microscopic implantation on peritoneum		
b	Limited to true pelvis with (-) nodes and implantation on peritoneum none greater than 2 cm		
c	Retroperitoneal or inguinal node involvement or abdominal implants greater than 2 cm		
IV	Distant metastasis; pleural effusions must contain malignant cells; liver involvement must be parenchymal.	5	0%

Staging Breast Cancer[114]

Stage	Tumor	Lymph nodes	Mets	TNM Class
0	Noninvasive carcinoma in situ; Paget's dz of nipple	(-) N_0	(-)	$T_{is}N_0M_0$
I	Greatest dimension $\leq$ 2cm (T_1)	(-) N_0	(-)	$T_1N_0M_0$
IIA	2 cm < Tumor $\leq$ 5 cm (T_2)	(+) ipsilateral but not fixed (N_1)	(-)	$T_{0-1}N_1M_0$ $T_2N_0M_0$
IIB	2cm < Tumor < 5+ cm (T_3)	(+) ipsilateral but not fixed (N_1)	(-)	$T_2N_1M_0$ $T_3N_0M_0$
IIIA	Tumor > 5 cm (T_3)	(+) ipsi, fixed to each other, skin, or chest wall (N_2)	(-)	$T_{0-2}N_2M_0$ $T_3N_{1-2}M_0$
IIIB	Any size (T_4) with: skin nodules or skin ulceration or fixation to skin/chest wall or breast edema incl. peau d'orange	Supra/infraclavicular LNs; edema of arm ± palpable axillary LNs (N_3)	(-)	$T_4N_{any}M_0$ $T_{any}N_3M_0$
IV	Any size	Any status	(+)	$T_{any}N_{any}M_1$

Axillary lymph nodes & survival

Axillary lymph nodes	5 years (%)	10 yrs (%)
None positive	80	65
1-3 nodes positive	65	40
> 3 nodes positive	30	15

Tumor size & survival

Tumor size	10 yrs (%)
< 1 cm	80
3-4 cm	55
5-7.5 cm	45

[113] Bast RC & Berchuck A, "Ovarian cancer," in JD Wilson *et al* (eds), *Harrison's Principles of Internal Medicine* 12/e 1991,NY:McGraw-Hill. American Joint Committee on Cancer, Beahrs OH (ed), *Manual for staging of cancer*, Philadelphia: JB Lippincott, 1992.
[114] American Joint Committee on Cancer, Beahrs OH (ed), *Manual for staging of cancer*, Philadelphia: JB Lippincott, 1992. DA Casciato & BA Lowitz, *Manual of Clinical Oncology*, 3/e, Boston: Little, Brown, 1995.

Survival by AJCC stage, based on 50,834 pts diagnosed 1983-7

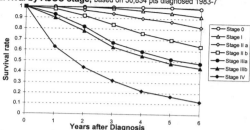

Estrogen receptor positivity: Confers a better prognosis

Node-Negative Breast Cancer[115]

Treatment: • 70% cured surgically without adjuvant therapy • Tamoxifen reduces recurrence ~25% (esp age > 50 ± menopause) • Polychemotherapy reduces recurrence ~30% (esp age < 60)

Tumor size & histopathological grade

Tumor Size	Proportion	5-year survival	20-yr recurrence
< 1 cm	8%	99%	14%
1 - 3 cm	64%	91%	31% (1-2cm)
> 3 cm	28%	85%	> 50%

Late recurrence<10%: ductal CA in situ; pure tubular; papillary; typical medullary
Nuclear and histologic grades: Unreliable in inexperienced hands: well-differentiated (Grade 1) good prognosis; consider sending-out test
Estrogen-receptor status
Predicts response to tamoxifen. ER+ only 8-10% disease-free survival benefit.
S-Phase fraction & ploidy: Aneuploid may have worse prognosis
  Low-S-phase fraction (slow-growing) have better disease-free survival; each
  laboratory must have validated cutoffs before results are used;
Cathepsin D: Lysosomal enzyme overexpressed in certain tumors, may have
  role in metastasis. Overexpression may be an ominous sign.

5-year recurrence according to various risk factors (%)

Ductal carcinoma in situ	2		Estrogen-receptor positive	25
Tumor < 1.0 cm	6		Aneuploid tumor	26
Nuclear grade 1	7		Nuclear grade 3	28
Low S-phase fraction	10		High S-phase fraction	30
Diploid tumor	12		Estrogen-receptor negative	34
Tumor = 1.1-20 cm	13		High cathepsin D level	50
Nuclear grade 2	24		Aneuploid, high cathepsin D	60

[115] WL McGuire, GM Clarke, "Prognostic factors and treatment decisions in axillary-node negative breast cancer," N Engl J Med, 326(26):1756, 1992.

Infectious Disease

Bacterial Endocarditis Prophylaxis[116]

Cardiac conditions for which prophylaxis IS recommended
• Prosthetic cardiac valves • Previous bacterial endocarditis • Most congenital cardiac malformations • Rheumatic and other acquired valve dysfunction, even after valve surgery • Hypertrophic cardiomyopathy • Mitral valve prolapse (only with mitral regurgitation)

Cardiac conditions for which prophylaxis NOT recommended
• Isolated secundum atrial septal defect • Surgical repair without residua beyond 6 months of isolated secundum ASD, VSD, or PDA • Previous CABG • Mitral valve prolapse without regurgitation (Risk may be increased with thickening/redundancy of leaflets, esp in men > 45 yrs) • Physiological or innocent heart murmurs • Previous Kawasaki disease without valvular dysfunction • Previous rheumatic fever without valvular dysfunction • Cardiac pacemakers & AICDs

Selected procedures for which prophylaxis IS recommended
• Dental procedures known to induce gingival bleeding (incl cleaning) • Tonsillectomy / adenoidectomy • Surgical procedures involving respiratory or gastrointestinal mucosa • Rigid bronchoscopy • Sclerotherapy for esophageal varices • Esophageal dilatation • Gallbladder surgery • Cystoscopy • Urethral dilatation • Urethral catheterization in presence of urinary tract infection* • Urinary tract surgery in presence of urinary tract infection* • Prostate surgery • Incision & drainage of infected tissue* • Vaginal hysterectomy • Vaginal delivery in the presence of infection*

Procedures for which prophylaxis is NOT recommended**
• Dental procedures unlikely to produce gingival bleeding • Local intraoral anesthetic injections except intraligamentary • Shedding of primary teeth • Tympanostomy tube insertion • Endotracheal intubation or Flexible bronchoscopy with or without biopsy • Cardiac catheterization • Endoscopy with or without biopsy • Cesarean delivery • In absence of infection: uretheral catheterization, dilatation and curettage, uncomplicated vaginal delivery, therapeutic abortion, sterilization procedure, insertion or removal of IUDs

Regimens for dental, oral, upper resp procedures in pts at risk
- **Standard:**
  - Amoxicillin 3 g po 1 hr before procedure and 1.5 g 6 hrs later
  - Unable to take po : Ampicillin 2 g IV/IM 30 min before procedure then 1 g IV/IM or amoxicillin 1.5 g po 6 hrs after first dose
  - "Very-high risk:" Ampicillin 2 g IV/IM plus gentamicin 1.5 mg/kg IV/IM (<80 mg) 30 min before procedure, followed by amoxicillin 1.5 g po 6 hrs later. Alternatively, give amp/gent 8 hrs after 1st

- **Penicillin-allergic:**
  - Erythromycin ethylsuccinate 800mg or stearate 1 g po 2 hrs before procedure and then ½ dose 6 hrs later;

---

[116] Dajani AS, *et al*, "Prevention of bacterial endocarditis," _JAMA_ 264:2919, 1990. Durack DT, "Prevention of infective endocarditis,"_N Engl J Med_ 1995;332(1):38-44.
* In addition to prophylactic regimen for GU procedure, therapy should be directed agianst most likely bacterial pathogen.
** In patients with prosthetic heart valves or previous history of endocarditis, physicians may elect prophylaxis even for low-risk procedures that involve the lower respiratory, GU, or GI tract.

- Or Clindamycin 300 mg po 1 hr before & 150 mg 6 hrs later
- Unable to take po: Clindamycin 300 IV 30 min pre & 150 mg IV/po 6 hrs post
- "Very high risk:" Vancomycin 1 g IV over 1 hr beginning 1 hr before procedure. No repeat dose necessary

Regimens for genitourinary and gastrointestinal procedures
- Low-risk: Amoxicillin 3 g po 1 hr before then 1.5 g 6 hrs later
- Standard: Ampicillin 2 g IV/IM plus gentamicin 1.5 mg/kg IV/IM (<80 mg) 30 min before, then amoxicillin 1.5 g po 6 hrs later. Alternatively repeat amp/gent 8 hrs after first.
- Pencillin-allergic: Vancomycin 1 g IV over 1 hr plus gentamicin 1.5 mg/kg IV/IM (<80mg) 1 hr before procedure. May repeat after 8 hrs.

Prophylaxis for cardiac surgery with foreign material placement
- Standard Cefazolin 2 g IV immediately preoperatively then q 6 hrs for 24-48 hrs plus gentamicin 1.7 mg/kg IV immediately preop and q 8 hrs x 24 hrs.
- At institutions with high incidence of MRSA: Vancomycin 15 mg/kg over 1 hr immediately preop then 10 mg/kg IV after CABG plus gentamicin as above.

Rheumatic Fever: Jones Criteria[117]

Major manifestations	Minor manifestations	Evidence of antecedent group A streptococcal infection[d]
Carditis[a]	Fever	Positive throat culture or rapid streptococcal antigen test
Polyarthritis[b]	Arthralgia	Elevated or rising streptococcal antibody titer
Sydenham's chorea	↑ ESR	
Erythema marginatum	↑ C-reactive protein	
SubQ nodules[c]	Prolonged PR interval	

a: almost always with murmur of valvulitis
b: almost always migratory unless aborted with NSAIDS, large joints, almost never deforming, almost always dramatic response to salicylates < 48h
c: over joint extensor surfaces, occiput, vertebral spinous processes
d: note streptococcal skin infections not associated with rheumatic fever

Diagnosis
If supported by evidence of antecedent group A streptococcal infection, the presence of two major manifestations or of one major and two minor manifestations indicates a high probability of acute rheumatic fever
Exceptions to Jones criteria: (1) Isolated chorea; (2) Indolent carditis (3) History of rheumatic fever with one major or two minor manifestations and evidence of recent group A strep infection

Routine Vaccines for Adults[118]

Vaccine	Indicated for	Dosage	Contraindicated	Adverse rxn
Tetanus-diphtheria (Adult Td)				
Adsorbed tetanus and diphtheria toxoids	Unimmunized	2 doses 0.5 ml IM 1-2 mo apart, 3rd dose 6-12mo later	Neuro reaaction or hypersensitivity to previous dose	Local pain and swelling (severe if given too often)
	Everyone	Boost q 10 yr		

[117] "Guidelines for the diagnosis of rheumatic fever: Jones Criteria, updated 1992," Circulation, 1993; 87(1):302.
[118] "Routine immunization for adults,"Medical Letter on Drugs and Therapeutics, 1990; 32(819):54-6.

Vaccine	Indicated for	Dosage	Contraindicated	Adverse rxn
Influenza				
Inactivated whole or virus subunits; chick embryo cells	High-risk pts, health-care workers; all > 65 yrs old	1 dose 0.5 ml IM annually	Egg allergy	Local soreness
Pneumococcal				
Capsular polysaccharides from 23 types	High-risk patients; all > 65 years old	1 dose 0.5 ml IM		Local soreness
Hepatitis B				
Recombinant hepatitis B surface antigen	High-risk patients and health-care workers	3 doses 1 ml IM deltoid, 2nd after 1 mo, 3rd 6 mo after 1st; higher dose for immune compromized & dialysis patients	None	Local soreness
Measles				
Attenuated live virus grown in chick fibroblasts	Unimmunized, born after 1956	2 doses 0.5 ml SQ at least one month apart	Egg allergy; neomycin hypersensitivity; pregnancy; immune compromise	Low-grade fever
	Previously immunized with 1 dose; college entry; health-care workers, foreign travel	1 dose 0.5 ml SQ		
Rubella				
Attenuated live virus, grown in human diploid cells (RA 27/3 strain)	Unimmunized young women and health care workers	1 dose 0.5 ml SQ	Pregnancy; immune compromise; hypersensitivity to neomycin	Low-grade fever, rash, LAN, sore throat, arthritis in up to 40% of nonimmune adults

Streptococcal Endocarditis Risk[119]

Probability of endocarditis if bacteremic with:

Bacterium	Endocarditis: Nonendocarditis	Bacterium	Endocarditis: Nonendocarditis
S. mutans	14.2:1	Misc streptococci	1:1.3
S. bovis	5.9:1	S. bovis II	1:1.7
Dextran-forming mitior	3.3:1	S. anginosus	1:2.6
S. Sanguis	3.0:1	Group G streptococci	1:2.9
S. mitior	1.8:1	Group B streptococci	1:7.4
Unclassified "viridans"	1.4:1	Group A streptococci	1:32.0
Enterococcus faecalis	1:1.2		

[119] Parker MT, Ball LC, "Streptococci and aerococci associated with systemic infection in man," J Med Microbiol, 1976;9:275-302.

Bacterial vs. Viral Meningitis[120]

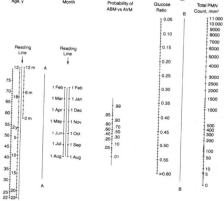

Nomogram for estimating probability of acute bacterial vs viral meningitis. **(1)** Place ruler on reading lines for pt age & month of presentation. Mark intersection on line A. **(2)** Repeat for glucose & CSF WBC count on line B. **(3)** Place ruler on the marks on lines A & B and read probability of bacterial vs viral meningitis. Derived from Duke data 1969-80. No prospective validation to date; a retrospective validation is published.[121]

Toxic Shock Syndrome

Diagnostic Criteria[122]:
- Temperature > 38.9°C • Systolic BP < 90 mm Hg for adults; postural diastolic BP ↓ 15 mm Hg; orthostatic syncope or dizziness
- Rash with subsequent desquamation 1-2 wks after onset, esp palms/soles
- Multiorgan involvement (at least 3 of following:) • GI: vomitting, profuse diarrhea • Musculoskeletal: severe myalgia, CPK ≥ fivefold increase • Mucosa (vagina, conjunctivae, pharynx): frank hyperemia • Renal: BUN or Cr > twice normal with pyuria (>5 WBC/hpf), not UTI • Hepatic: T. Bili or transaminase > twice upper normal limit • Hematologic: Platelets < 100,000 • CNS: Disorientation, alteration in consciousness without focal signs when fever and hypotension are absent

[120] Spanos, *et al*, "Differential diagnosis of acute meningitis: an analysis of the predictive value of initial observations," <u>JAMA</u> 262(19):2700-7, 1989. Copyright 1989, American Medical Association, reproduced with permission.
[121] McKinney WP *et al*, "Validation of a clinical prediction rule for the differential diagnosis of acute meningitis," <u>J Gen Intern Med</u> 1994; 9:8-12.
[122] Reingold AL, *et al*, "Toxic shock syndrome surveillance in the US, 1980-1," <u>Ann Intern Med</u> 1982; 96:875.

- Negative cultures of blood (except *S aureus*), pharynx, & CSF; No rise in titer to agents of Rocky Mountain spotted fever, leptospira, rubeola

Differential diagnosis

- Rocky Mountain spotted fever • Meningococcemia • Drug reactions / erythema multiforme / Stephens Johnson • Kawasaki disease • Streptococcal infection including Scarlet fever (may be indistinguishable) • Staphylococcal scalded skin syndrome • Septic shock • Viral exanthems

Common clinical manifestations[123]

SYMPTOMS	%
Myalgia	92
Vomitting	90
Diarrhea	86
Headache	72
Dizziness	70
Sore throat	65
SIGNS	**%**
Abd. Tenderness	83
Pharyngitis / strawberry tongue	81
Peripheral edema	73
Conjunctivitis	65
CNS dysfunction	60
Vaginal inflammation	47

LABS	%
↑ WBC	70
↑ PT	70
Anemia (1st 24h)	66
↓ Platelets	52
↑ PTT	
↓ Albumin, Ca	81, 80
↑ AST	73
↑ Cr, BUN	69, 68
↑ T. bilirubin	66
↑ CPK	66
↓ Phosphorus	60
Pyuria	77
Hematuria	46

Infections after Transplantation[124]

Timing of common infections after marrow transplant

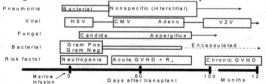

Viral infections after Marrow transplant

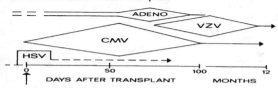

[123] Parsonnet J, Kasper DL, "Toxic shock syndrome: clinical developments and new biology," in Wilson JD *et al* (eds), <u>Harrison's Principles of Internal Medicine, supplement 1,</u> 1992.

Severe infections after liver transplant (Episodes per pt/year)

Time after transplant (mo)	1	2	3	4-6	7-12	>12
All infections	7.1	4.5	1.0	0.9	0.3	0.2
Bacterial	4.4	1.6	0.7	0.5	0.3	0.2
Fungal	1.3	0.66	0	0.05	0.02	0
Viral	1.2	2.0	0	0.05	0	0
Protozoal (mostly PCP)	0.24	0.26	0.28	0.30	0	0

Solid-organ transplant infections in the first year:

Type	Infection per pt	Infection mortality	Bacter-emia	Symptom-atic CMV	Invasive fungus	Site most common
Renal n=64	0.98	0	5%	5%	0	UTI 41%
Heart n=119	1.36	15%	13%	5%	8%	Lung 27%
Heart-Lung n=31	3.19	45%	19%	32%	23%	Lung 57%
Liver n=101	1.86	23%	23%	5%	16%	Abd,GI 23%

Occupational HIV Exposure[125]

Risk of HIV infection after percutaneous exposure

- Average risk: 0.3%
- Increased risk from (1) deep injury; (2) visible blood on device causing injury; (3) device previously placed in the source-patient's vein or artery, (4) source-patient who died of AIDS within 60 days postexposure, presumably having high HIV titer.
- Mucous membrane exposure to HIV-infected blood: 0.1%
- Skin exposure to HIV-infected blood: <0.1%

Initiate postexposure prophylaxis promptly, preferably within 1-2 hrs.

Type of Exposure	Source Material	Antiretroviral prophylaxis[a]	Antiretroviral regimen[b]
Percutaneous	**Blood**[c]		
	Highest risk	Recommend	ZDV + 3TC + IDV
	Increased risk	Recommend	ZDV + 3TC ± IDV[d]
	No increased risk	Offer	ZDV + 3TC
	"Infectious" fluid[e]	Offer	ZDV + 3TC
	Other fluid (eg urine)	Not offer	
Mucous membrane	**Blood**[c]	Offer	ZDV + 3TC ± IDV[d]
	"Infectious" fluid[e]	Offer	ZDV + 3TC
	Other fluid (eg urine)	Not offer	
Skin[f], increased risk	**Blood**[c]	Offer	ZDV + 3TC ± IDV[d]
	"Infectious" fluid[e]	Offer	ZDV ± 3TC
	Other fluid (eg urine)	Not offer	

a: Recommend (Offer): Postexposure prophylaxis (PEP) should be recommended (or offered) to the exposed worker with counseling. Not offer: PEP should not be offered because these are not occupational exposures to HIV.

124 JD Meyers, "Infections in marrow transplant recipients," and M Ho et al "Infections in solid organ transplant recipients," in in Mandell, Douglass, Bennett, (eds), Principles and practice of infectious disease, 3rd, New York: Churchill-Livingstone, 1990. Reproduced with permission.
125 "Provisional Public Health Service recommendations for chemoprophylaxis after occupational exposure to HIV," Morbidity & Mortality Weekly Report, 1996;45(22):468-472.

b: Regimens: zidovudine (ZDV) 200 mg tid, lamivudine (3TC) 150 mg bid, indinavir (IDV) 800 mg tid. If IDV is not available, saquinavir may be used, 600 mg tid. Prophylaxis is given for 4 weeks.

c: Highest risk: BOTH larger volume of blood (eg deep injury with large-bore hollow needle previously in source-patient's blood vessel, especially involving injection of source-patient blood) AND blood containing a high-titer of HIV (eg source-patient with acute retroviral illness or end-stage AIDS. **Increased risk**: EITHER large-volume exposure OR high-titer HIV. **No increased risk**: NEITHER of above (eg solid suture needle injury from source-patient with asymptomatic HIV infection).

d: Possible toxicity of additional drug may not be warranted.

e: Infectious fluid: Fluid containing visible blood, semen, vaginal secretions, CSF, synovial, pleural, peritoneal, pericardial, amniotic fluids.

f: For skin, risk is increased for exposures involving a high titer of HIV, prolonged contact, an extensive area, or an area in which skin integrity is visibly compromised. For skin exposures without increased risk, the risk for drug toxicity outweighs the benefit of postexposure prophylaxis.

Resistance to specific antiretroviral agents
- More likely if source-patient used agent > 6-12 mo, if source-patient complied poorly with the drug regimen, if viral replication was not completely suppressed in the source-patient, and in increased viral replication during advanced HIV-infection (eg CD4+ count < 200 cells/mm³).
- Consider adding a protease inhibitor for lower-risk exposures if ZDV-resistant strains are likely.
- If there is suspicion that source-patient has a resistant HIV strain, follow PHS recommendations initially and then seek expert consultation to construct an alternative regimen. Generally these will include two nucleoside analogues plus a protease inhibitor or nevirapine.

Neurology

Early Management of Stroke[126]

Initial Assessment: Determine if stroke is _ischemic_ or _hemorrhagic_
- **General medical: ♦** Frequent vital signs ♦ Head or neck trauma;
  - ♦ Cardiovascular abnormalities; ♦ Ocular signs
- **Neurological exam: ♦** Level of consciousness ♦ Glasgow coma scale score 3-15 ♦ Pupils ♦ Individual limb movements ♦ Meningeal signs
- Urgent CT of the brain without contrast
  - ♦ Emergency ultrasound when suspicion of symptomatic carotid disease
  - ♦ LP if strong suspicion of subarachnoid hemorrhage and (-) CT
  - ♦ Lateral cervical spine roentgenogram in comatose patients or those with cervical spine pain or tenderness
- ECG, CXR, CBC, Platelets, PT, aPTT, electrolytes, glucose, ABG

General treatment considerations
- ♦ Ensure adequate airway   ♦ Avoid hypotonic fluids

---

126 McDowell FH, et al, "Stroke: the first six hours. National Stroke Association consensus statement," <u>Stroke Clinical Updates</u>, 1993; 4(1):1; "Guidelines for cardiopulmonary resuscitation and emergency care," <u>JAMA</u> 1992; 268:2171-2302.

♦ If seizures occur, administer ♦ **Phenytoin** 15 mg/kg orally or IV, given no faster than 50 mg/min IV ♦ **Diazepam** 10 mg IV ♦ **Phenobarbital** 15 mg/kg IV; cautious observation for respiratory depression.

♦ Do not treat elevated BP unless sustained SBP>220 or DBP>120 or other indications (eg myocardial ischemia) or SAH (below)

♦ Increased intracranial pressure: ♦ Fluid restriction ♦ Mannitol (1-2g/kg IV over 5-10 min) ♦ Consider intubation and hyperventilation to a P_aCO_2 of 25-28 torr ♦ Consider intraventricular catheter CSF drainage ♦ Surgery

Acute ISCHEMIC stroke

♦ If cerebellar infarction, consult neurosurgeon.
♦ If brainstem infarction, consider urgent surgical decompression.
♦ If discrete onset < 180 min consider tPA (see page 123).

Acute SUBARACHNOID HEMORRHAGE

♦ Consult neurosurgeon. ♦ Lower BP to estimated prestroke levels ♦ Nimodipine 60 mg po q 6hr if patient not stuporous ♦ Analgesics and sedatives as needed
♦ Urgent angiography, invasive hemodynamic monitoring with consideration of early surgery in aneurysmal SAH

Acute INTRACEREBRAL HEMORRHAGE

♦ Consult neurosurgeon in cerebellar hemorrhage or acute hydrocephalus

Therapeutic options not yet established

♦ Intravenous heparin in nonhemorrhagic stroke
♦ Intraarterial or systemic thrombolytics in nonhemorrhagic stroke guided by arteriography or transcranial ultrasound
♦ Aspirin or ticlopidine in acute stroke
♦ Early craniotomy/stereotaxy for intracranial hemorrhage.
♦ Urgent surgery for aneurysmal subarachnoid hemorrhage

Status Epilepticus[127]

Definition: Seizures > 30 min or sequential without intercurrent return to neurologic baseline.

Etiologies:

♦ Structural: Brain trauma, tumor, stroke, hemorrhage
♦ CNS infection: encephalitis, meningitis
♦ Toxic: Drugs: penicillins, lidocaine, normeperidine, theophylline, flumazenil, cocaine, imipenem
♦ Drug withdrawal: EtOH, opiates, barbiturates, benzodiazepines
♦ Metabolic: ↓ Glucose; ↑ glucose; ↓ sodium; ↓ calcium; ↓ magnesium; ↑ osmolarity; hypoxia; uremia
♦ Precipitation of idiopathic epilepsy: Change in anticonvulsant drug levels (drug interactions, noncompliance, altered absorption); Intercurrent infection; EtOH excess or withdrawal

Management: STOP the SEIZURE

♦ Assure adequate airway, intubate as warranted
♦ Establish IV access; Phlebotomy: CBC/diff, Chem-7+ Ca, Mg, anticonvulsant levels, tox screen; D50 + Thiamine; Monitor VS, EKG

Administer Drugs sequentially until the seizure is aborted:
♦ **Lorazepam** 0.1 mg/kg IV < 2 mg/min
  ♦ Compared to diazepam, slower onset (2 min vs 15 sec) but no rebound seizures from redistribution from CNS to peripheral tissues. Both have disadvantage of delaying phenytoin if only single IV available

127 C Phillips & AM Blumenfeld, "Status epilepticus," in JM Rippe et al (eds.), Intensive Care Medicine, 2/e, Boston: Little, Brown & Co., 1991.

- ◆ **OR Diazepam** 5-10 mg IV (give same formulation **per rectum** if no IV access)
- ◆ **Phenytoin** 20 mg/kg IV not faster than 50 mg/min, slower for hypotension
  - ◆ Rebolus 5 mg/kg to maximum total 30 mg/kg if still seizing
- ◆ **Phenobarbital** 20 mg/kg not faster than 100 mg/min   ◆ Intubate
- ◆ **Pentobarbital** 5 mg/kg load → 5 mg/kg prn until EEG burst-suppression (intermittent mixed-frequency pattern with flat background) → 0.5-2 mg/kg/hr
  - ◆ EEG q 1-2 hr to ensure burst-suppression pattern remains
  - ◆ Stop infusion at 12 hrs; if seizures recur, resume infusion for longer periods
  - ◆ Consider inhalational anesthetics, benzodiazepine infusion

Delirium Tremens[128]

Manifestations: Typically 72-96 hours after cessation of drinking
- ◆ Autonomic instability, tremulousness, agitation, diaphoresis, nausea
- ◆ Hallucinosis: Visual > auditory; Unlike schizophrenia, pts attempt to respond appropriately.
- ◆ Seizure: Typically generalized, herald DT 1/3 cases; focal seizures suggest CNS lesions
- ◆ Mortality high as 15%. Related to complications: VT, pneumonia, sepsis, electrolytes...

Differential diagnosis
- ◆ Withdrawal: Minor alcohol (8-48hrs); Narcotics; Barbiturates
- ◆ Metabolic disorders: (1) **Wernicke** Encephalopathy: Ataxia, Confusion, Opthalmopathy (usually bilat. nystagmus); (2) **Electrolytes**: Magnesium, sodium, phosphorus, hyperosmolar states, hypoglycemia; (3) **Ingestions**: drugs, antifreeze; (4) **Hepatic encephalopathy**; (5) **Uremia**; (6) **Hypoxia**; (7) **Hypothermia**
- ◆ Neurological emergencies: (1) **Hypertensive encephalopathy**: Funduscopic exam essential; (2) **Intracerebral hemorrhage**; (3) **Meningitis/Encephalitis**; (3) **Postictal** state or temporal seizures   ◆ Endocrine: Hypoglycemia; Thyroid storm   ◆ Psychosis, organic or drug-mediated   ◆ Sepsis

Special Exams
- ◆ Eyes: fundus, nystagmus;   ◆ Neck: Thyroid, meningismus;
- ◆ Chvostek/Trousseau signs;   ◆ Liver disease stigmata;   ◆ Focal neurological findings;   ◆ Cognitive exam;   ◆ Evidence of trauma

Management
- ◆ Monitor in ICU if requires restraints, if severe metabolic derangements, if concurrent moderate-severe infection
- ◆ Benzodiazepines vs clonidine vs phenobarbital   ◆ Intractable seizures: phenytoin, paraldehyde
- ◆ Correct electrolytes   ◆ Restraints if threat of self-injury   ◆ Antipyretics   ◆ Thiamine & Folate

Other alcohol-related syndromes & complications
- ◆ Neuro: Korsakoff's psychosis, cerebellar degeneration, central pontine myelinolysis, polyneuropathy   ◆ Rhabdomyolysis & cardiomyopathy   ◆ Hepatitis, gastritis, pancreatitis   ◆ Ketoacidosis & Nutritional deficiencies   ◆ Hypogonadism

---

[128] "Alcohol withdrawal syndrome." N Engl J Med 1985; 313:951-2. "Alcohol withdrawal symptoms." J Gen Intern Med 1989;4:432-44. "Alcoholism." Ann Intern Med 1984;100:405-16. "Life-threatening ventricular ventricular tachyarrhythmias in delirium tremens." Arch Intern Med 1977; 137:1238.

Cerebrospinal Fluid Data

Total protein in CSF from 4200 patients[129]

Diagnosis	CSF protein range (mg/dL); Percent of patients with each disease					Average (mg/dL)
	< 45	45-75	75-100	100-500	>500	
Purulent meningitis	2	4	8	64	22	418
Aseptic meningitis	46	25	9	21	-	77
Brain abscess	27	45	9	18	-	69
TB meningitis	1	12	15	68	5	200
Neurosyphilis	46	29	11	13	-	68
Acute EtOH	92	6	2	-	-	32
Uremia	58	25	15	2	-	57
Myxedema	24	55	6	16	-	71
Epilepsy (idiopathic)	90	10	-	-	-	31
Brain tumor	31	25	12	31	1	115
Cord tumor	14	11	8	39	28	425
Cerebral trauma	54	18	9	15	4	100
Multiple sclerosis	68	24	6	3	-	43
Polyneuritis	51	16	8	21	5	74
Poliomyelitis	47	28	10	15	-	70
Cerebral thrombosis	66	26	4	3	-	46
Cerebral hemorrhage	14	17	13	38	18	270

Hypoglycorrhachia syndromes (CSF/serum glucose < 0.5)
◆ Acute bacterial meningitis ◆ TB meningitis ◆ Fungal meningitis ◆ Carcinomatous meningitis ◆ Meningeal sarcoidosis ◆ Amebic & helminthic meningitis: *Naegleria, Cysticerca, Trichinella* ◆ Acute syphilitic meningitis & generalized paresis ◆ Subarachnoid hemorrhage ◆ Chemical meningitis after intrathecal infusion, myelogram, spinal anesthesia, etc. ◆ Specific viruses: lymphocytic choriomeningitis, mumps, uncommonly in herpes simplex/zoster meningitis ◆ Hypoglycemia ◆ Rheumatoid meningitis ◆ SLE myelopathy

Initial CSF findings in ~150 pts with PURULENT meningitis[130]

	Meningo-coccus	Pneumo-coccus	Strepto-coccus	Staphylo-coccus	H influenza	Percent
Cells/mm³						
< 100	1	0	0	1	0	1
100-1000	5	3	1	2	1	12
1,000-10,000	39	31	27	8	4	72
10k-20,000	11	2	2	1	0	10
> 20,000	6	0	1	1	0	5
Protein (mg/dL)						
< 45	1	0	1	1	0	2
45-100	7	2	7	3	0	12
100-500	39	29	23	4	5	64
500-1000	7	6	8	1	0	14
1000-2000	10	3	0	0	0	8

---

[129] HH Merritt & F Fremont-Smith, <u>The Cerebrospinal Fluid</u>, Philadelphia: Saunders, 1938. Cited in RA Fishman, <u>Cerebrospinal fluid in diseases of the nervous system</u>, 2/e, p 200, Philadelphia: Saunders, 1992. Adapted with permission.
[130] RA Fishman, *ibid*, p 259. Adapted with permission.

	Meningo-coccus	Pneumo-coccus	Strepto-coccus	Staphylo-coccus	*H influenza*	Percent
Glucose (mg/dL)						
< 10	13	12	8	0	2	23
10-40	38	19	19	8	3	57
40-50	2	3	3	2	0	6
50-60	5	1	4	0	1	7
60	3	2	5	1	0	7

Lumbar fluid changes in Brain Abscess[131]

Pressure (99 pts)	< 200	38%
	200-300	35%
	> 300	26%

Protein (mg/dL)	< 50	29%
	50-100	38%
	> 100	33%

WBC's (per mm³)	<5	29%
	5-100	38%
	> 100	33%

Glucose (mg/dL)	> 40	79%
	< 40	21%

Admission CSF findings in 35 pts with TB meningitis[132]

WBCs (per mm³)		Total	Died
	< 50	3	1
	51-200	12	2
	201-1,000	19	7
	> 1,000	1	1

Glucose (mg/dL)		Total	Died
	0-20	14	5
	21-40	12	4
	41-60	7	1
	> 60	2	1

PMNs (%)		Total	Died
	0	5	2
	1-25	20	5
	26-50	5	1
	51-75	4	3
	> 75	1	0

Protein (mg/dL)		Total	Died
	0-50	5	3
	21-100	7	1
	101-200	13	4
	> 200	10	3

AFB Smear		Total	Died
	+	7	1
	-	25	10
	Unknown	3	0

TB culture		Total	Died
	+	26	8
	-	8	3
	Unknown	1	0

Competency[133]

Components ◆Level of <u>arousal</u> must be adequate ◆Must be able to <u>comprehend</u> basic info relevant to competency, eg nature of illness, reasons for treatment, who are caregivers ◆Must be able to <u>retain</u> info long enough to consider in light of relevant experience. Written documents may help compensate. ◆If above elements intact, <u>judgement</u> and <u>awareness</u> must be adequate.

Attention ◆"Drifting:" Arousable but somnolent. Usually subcortical focal reticular system abnormality. Must be considered incompetent, even though otherwise intact when aroused. ◆"Wandering:" Easily distracted though adequately aroused; unable to maintain fixed direction. Thalamic projections; usually metabolic or toxic dysfunction. Competency depends on adequacy of attention span; typically 1 minute. Test calculation ability.

Language ◆Spontaneous speech: Aphasia (paraphasias, word-finding) does

[131] *Ibid*, p 270. Adapted with permission.
[132] AR Hinman, "Tuberculous meningitis at Cleveland Metropolitan General Hospital, 1959-63," *Am Rev Respir Dis*. 1967;95:670-3. With permssion, Amercan College of Chest Physicians. Cited in Fishman, *ibid*, p 272. Adapted with permission.
[133] Freedman et al, "Assessment of competency: the role of neurobehavioral deficits," *Ann Intern Med*, 1991;115:203.

not imply incompetence. Communicate by other means. ◆ Auditory: Incompetent if unable to understand single words or phrases. Test logical and consistent responses on repeated assessment. ◆ Reading comprehension: Usually parallels impaired auditory comprehension. May be improved by having pt read aloud. ◆ Writing: Assess if pt unable to speak

Memory ◆ Recent and remote may be dissociated, eg in Wernicke's or anterior communicating artery rupture

Frontal lobe dysfunction ◆ Awareness: ◆ Test awareness of family & social activities, emotional changes, levels of interest; compare with info from family. ◆ Discrepancies between what pt reports and what pt demonstrates. ◆ Judgement: inability to consider implications of facts and events. ◆ Impulsivity, goal selection, consistency of performance.

Hypoxic-Ischemic Coma: Prognosis[134]

Patients with virtually no chance of regaining independence

Initial	No pupillary light response
1 d	Motor response no better than flexor and spontaneous eye movements neither orienting nor roving-conjugate.
3 d	3-day motor response no better than flexor.
1 wk	1-wk motor not obeying commands & initial spont. eye movem'ts neither orienting nor roving conjugate & 3-day eye opening not spontaneous.
2 wk	2-week oculocephalic response not normal and 3-day motor response not obeying commands and 3-day eye opening not spontaneous and 2-week eye opening not improved at least two grades (none < other < roving-dysconj < roving-conj < orienting)

Patients with best chance of regaining independence

Initial	Pupillary light reflexes present & motor response flexor/extensor & spontaneous eye movements roving-conjugate or orienting.
1 d	1-day motor response withdrawal or better and 1-day eye opening improved at least 2 grades
3 d	3d motor response withdrawal+ and 3d spontaneous eye movements normal.
1 wk	1-week motor response obeying commands.
2 wk	2-week oculocephalic response normal.

Rules based on neuro exam: **Coma** = no eye opening regardless of stimulus, no comprehensible words; commands not obeyed. **Vegetative state** = eyes open to noise or to pain, but no comprehensible words; commands not obeyed. **Conscious** = Comprehensible words or commands obeyed.

Outcome categories: (A)=No recovery, persistent vegetative state; (B)=Severe disability; (C)=Moderate disability, good recovery

	Best 1-year recovery (% total)		
106 Comatose pts at day 1	A	B	C
(1) 1d Spont. eye movement roving-conjugate or better	63	16	21
(2) Not (1) and Initial motor: withdrawal or better	82	0	14
(3) Not (2) and 1d oculovestibular any response	100	0	0
(4) Not (3)	98	0	2
47 Vegetative pts at day 1			
(1) 1d motor withdrawal or better	38	19	42
(2) Not (1) & 1d Spont eye movement any roving or better		18	0
(3) Not (2)		0	0

[134] D Levy, et al, "Predicting outcome from hypoxic-ischemic coma," JAMA 1985;253(10):1420.

15 Conscious pts at day 1	Best 1-year recovery (% total)		
(1) Initial pupillary reflex present & 1d spontaneous eye mov't roving-conjugate or better & oculovestibular normal	0	0	100
(2) Not (1)	86	0	14

Spinal & Peripheral Nerves[135]

Anterior aspect: Peripheral segments on left; Spinal segments on right

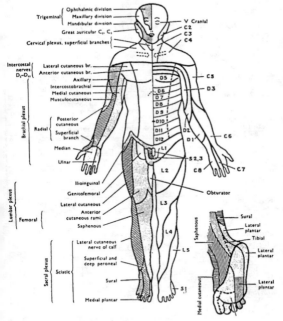

[135] J. Walton (ed.), <u>Brain's diseases of the nervous system</u>, 10/e, Oxford: Oxford University Press, 1993, p 47, by permission of Oxford University Press.

Posterior aspect: Spinal segments on left; Peripheral on right

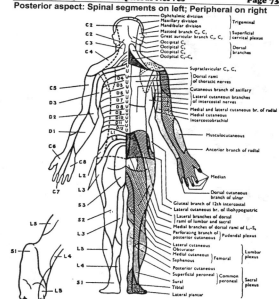

Labels (peripheral, right side):
- Ophthalmic division ⎤
- Maxillary division ⎬ Trigeminal
- Mandibular division ⎦
- Mastoid branch C₂, C₃ ⎤ Superficial
- Great auricular branch C₂, C₃ ⎦ cervical plexus
- Occipital C₃ ⎤
- Occipital C₄ ⎬ Dorsal branches
- Occipital C₅ ⎮
- Occipital C₆-C₈ ⎦
- Supraclavicular C₃, C₄
- Dorsal rami of thoracic nerves
- Cutaneous branch of axillary
- Lateral cutaneous branches of intercostal nerves
- Medial and lateral cutaneous br. of radial
- Medial cutaneous
- Intercostobrachial
- Musculocutaneous
- Anterior branch of radial
- Median
- Dorsal cutaneous branch of ulnar
- Gluteal branch of 12th intercostal
- Lateral cutaneous br. of iliohypogastric
- Lateral branches of dorsal rami of lumbar and sacral
- Medial branches of dorsal rami of L₁-S₅ ⎤ Pudendal plexus
- Perforating branch of posterior cutaneous ⎦
- Lateral cutaneous
- Obturator ⎤
- Medial cutaneous ⎬ Femoral ⎤ Lumbar plexus
- Saphenous ⎦
- Posterior cutaneous
- Superficial peroneal ⎤ Common peroneal ⎤ Sacral plexus
- Sural
- Tibial
- Lateral plantar

Spinal segment labels (left side): C2, C2, C3, C4, C5, D3, D2, D1, C6, C8, C7, L2, L3, S3, S2, L3, L5, S1, L4, L5
(trunk): D3, D4, D5, D6, D7, D8, D9, D10, D11, D12, L1

Spinal root lesions

Root	Pain/Sensory Loss	Weakness	Reflex loss
C6	Digits 1 & 2, radial forearm	Biceps	Biceps
C7	Digits 2 & 3	Triceps	Triceps
C8	Digits 4 & 5, ulnar forearm	Wrist extensors, intrinsics of hand	None
L4	Anterior shin	Quadriceps	Knee jerk
L5	Lateral calf, medial foot	Toe extensors	None
S1	Posterior calf, lateral foot	Gastrocnemius	Ankle jerk

Visual Acuity Screen[136]

96

20/800

873

20/400

2 8 4 3		O X X	20/200
6 3 8 5 2		X O O	20/100
8 7 4 5 9		O X O	20/70
6 3 9 2 5		X O X	20/50
4 2 8 3 6 5		o X o	20/40
3 7 4 2 5 8		X X o	20/30
9 3 7 8 2 6		X o o	20/25

Hold card in good light 14 inches from eye. Record vision for each eye separately with and without glasses. Presbyopic patients should read through bifocal glasses. Myopic patients should wear glasses only.

Pupil Diameter (mm)

. ② ③ ④ ⑤ ⑥ ⑦ ⑧ ⑨

136136 Adapted with permission from J.G. Rosenbaum MD, Pocket Vision Screen, Beachwood, Ohio.

Folstein Mini-Mental State[137]

Orientation	5 points	Year, Season, Date, Day, Month
	5 points	State, County, Town, Hospital, Floor
Registration	3 points	Patient recites three consecutive objects named (eg, ball, flag, tree)
Attention, Calculation	5 points	Serial 7's (5 responses); Alternatively spell "WORLD" backwards
Recall	3 points	Three objects registered above
Language	2 points	Name a pencil watch
	1 point	Repeat "No ifs, ands, or buts."
	3 points	3-stage command: "Take a paper in your right hand, fold it in half, and put it on the floor."
	1 point	Read and obey, "Close your eyes."
	1 point	Write a sentence
	1 point	Copy design below
Level of consciousness	0 points	Assess along continuum: Alert-Drowsy-Stuporous-Comatose

CLOSE YOUR EYES

Score 0-23 suggests cognitive dysfunction, as does score 23-29 along with altered mental status.   Note 1/3 patients have no identifiable pathology.

Glasgow Coma Scale[138]

Best Motor Response	Obeys	6
	Localizes	5
	Withdraws	4
	Abnormal flexion	3
	Extends	2
	Nil	1
Verbal Response	Oriented	5
	Confused conversation	4
	Inappropriate words	3
	Incomprehensible sounds	2
	Nil	1

Eye Opening	Spontaneous	4
	To speech	3
	To pain	2
	Nil	1

Score	Mortality in Head Injury
3-5	>60%
6-8	12%
9-12	2%

[137] MF Folstein et al, "Mini-mental state: a practical method for grading the cognitive state of patients for the clinician," J Psychiatric Res 1975;12:189.
[138] GM Teasdale, B Jennet, "Assessment of coma and impaired consciousness: a practical scale," Lancet, 1974;2(872):81-4. Jennett B, et al, "Predicting outcome in individual patients after severe head injury," Lancet, 1976;17968):1031-4.

Pulmonary

Pulmonary Function Testing[139]

Spirometry in a healthy individual.

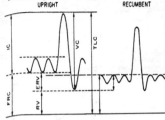

UPRIGHT   RECUMBENT

Abbreviations

ERV=expiratory reserve volume; $FEF_{25-75\%}$=forced expiratory flow from 25-75% vital capacity, an index of "small airways" obstruction; FEV_1= forced expiratory volume in 1s; FRC=functional residual capacity; FVC=forced vital capacity; IC=inspiratory capacity; MVV=maximum voluntary ventilation; RV= residual volume; TLC=total lung capacity; VC=vital capacity;

Disease Patterns

Obstructive: Resistance to outflow prolongs expiration. Therefore, $FEV_1/FVC < 70\%$; $FEF_{25-75\%}$ reduced, RV increased, MVV reduced, airway resistance ↑.

Restrictive: Reduced volumes without airways resistance. Therefore, VC ↓, FEV_1/FVC ↓ proportionately, MVV may be normal. Lung volumes should be confirmed by He-dilution or whole-body plethysmography. Differential diagnosis: interstitial dz, CHF, pneumonia, neuromuscular dz, chest wall abnormalities.

"Poor-effort" pattern: ↓VC, normal expiratory flow rates, ↓ MVV. Uneven, slurred, or notched spirometric curves and poor reproducibility.

Bronchodilator response: Predicts response to inhaled steroids & anticholinergics. Positive if 15% ↑ FVC increases 15% (at least 200cc); FEV_1 increases 12%; $FEF_{25-75\%}$ increases 25%.

Maximum minute ventilation (normal ~ 40×FEV_1) proportionately ↓ in obstruction but preserved until late interstitial dz. MVV generally should exceed 50% predicted before lung resection.

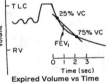

Expired Volume vs Time

Flow-Volume Loop

---

[139] John Leland Johnson, University Hospitals of Cleveland, Morning Rounds, March 20, 1992.

Quantitative severity of pulmonary impairment (% predicted)

Impairment	VC	FEV₁	FEV/FVC	FEF₂₅₋₇₅	TLC	DL_co
Normal	> 80	> 80	> 70	> 65	> 80	> 80
Mild	66-80	66-80	60-70	50-65	66-80	61-80
Moderate	50-65	50-65	45-59	35-49	50-65	40-60
Severe	< 50	< 50	< 45	< 35	< 50	< 40

Spirometry in obstructive & restrictive lung disease[140]

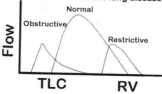

Mechanical upper airway obstruction

- Spirometric indices suggesting UAO: $FEV_1(ml) / PEFR (L/min) > 10$; $FEV_1/FEV_{0.5} > 1.5$; $MMV (L/min) / FEV_1 (L) < 25$.
- Variable extrathoracic: Bilateral or unilateral vocal cord paralysis, RA, post-intubation vocal cord adhesions, obstructive sleep apnea, burns.
- Variable intrathoracic: Localized non-circumferential tracheal tumors which make walls "floppy," relapsing polychondritis, tracheomalacia following surgery, mainstem bronchus tumors.
- Fixed upper airway obstruction: Benign stricture after prolonged intubation, tracheal tumor, goiter, small endotracheal or tracheostomy tube, bilateral stenosis of mainstem bronchi (rare).

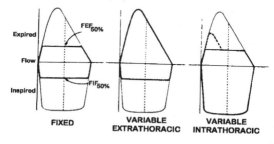

Chest Anatomy - Radiographs[141]

Posteroanterior Chest View

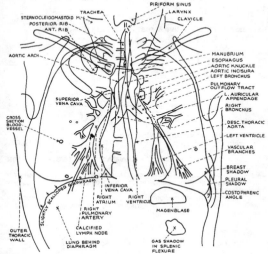

Azygos Lobe

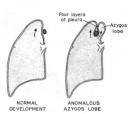

NORMAL DEVELOPMENT   ANOMALOUS AZYGOS LOBE

---

[141] I Meschan, <u>Roentgen signs in diagnostic imaging,</u> 2nd, 1987:Saunders, pp 4.72, 4.57, 4.82, 4.49. Reproduced with permission.

Lateral Chest View

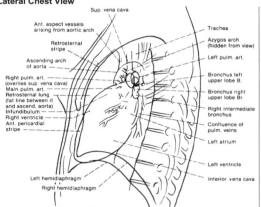

Sup. vena cava

Ant. aspect vessels arising from aortic arch

Retrosternal stripe

Ascending arch of aorta

Right pulm. art. (overlies sup. vena cava)
Main pulm. art.
Retrosternal lung (fat line between it and ascend. aorta)
Infundibulum
Right ventricle
Ant. pericardial stripe

Trachea

Azygos arch (hidden from view)

Left pulm. art.

Bronchus left upper lobe B.

Bronchus right upper lobe Br.

Right intermediate bronchus

Confluence of pulm. veins

Left atrium

Left ventricle

Inferior vena cava

Left hemidiaphragm
Right hemidiaphragm

Cardiac structures on PA chest radiograph

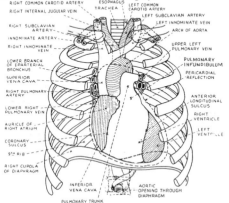

RIGHT COMMON CAROTID ARTERY
RIGHT INTERNAL JUGULAR VEIN
ESOPHAGUS
TRACHEA
LEFT COMMON CAROTID ARTERY
LEFT SUBCLAVIAN ARTERY
LEFT INNOMINATE VEIN
ARCH OF AORTA

RIGHT SUBCLAVIAN ARTERY
INNOMINATE ARTERY
RIGHT INNOMINATE VEIN

UPPER LEFT PULMONARY VEIN

PULMONARY INFUNDIBULUM
PERICARDIAL REFLECTION

LOWER BRANCH OF EPARTERIAL BRONCHUS
SUPERIOR VENA CAVA

RIGHT PULMONARY ARTERY

LOWER RIGHT PULMONARY VEIN

AURICLE OF RIGHT ATRIUM

CORONARY SULCUS

9 TH RIB

RIGHT CUPOLA OF DIAPHRAGM

ANTERIOR LONGITUDINAL SULCUS
RIGHT VENTRICLE
LEFT VENTRICLE

INFERIOR VENA CAVA

PULMONARY TRUNK

AORTIC OPENING THROUGH DIAPHRAGM

Chest Anatomy - CT[142]

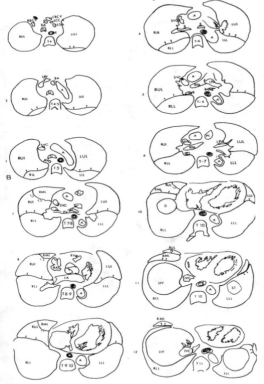

142 | Meschan, Roentgen signs in diagnostic imaging, 2nd, 1987: Saunders, p 4.49. Reproduced with permission.

Preoperative Pulmonary Testing[143]

Risk factors for poor outcome
- Airflow obstruction: • FEV1/FVC 55-70% mild; 40-55% mod; 25-40% severe; <25% extreme relative risk • FEV1 < 1 liter • MVV < 50% (reflects total effort)
- CO_2 retention, reflects decreased respiratory reserve
- Hypoxemia pO2<50 **unreliable**, may reflect shunting from surgical dz
- Pulmonary hypertension
- Site/type of operation: • Thoracotomy (sternotomy less than lateral thoracotomy) • Abdominal, upper>lower, muscle transection worst • Emergency (aspiration and no preoperative pulmonary optimization)
- Tobacco, especially age>40 • Recent infection • Obesity
- Age > 70 • Cooperation with pulmonary toilet.

Perioperative preparation
- Chronic (weeks before surgery): PFT's; Smoking cessation > 72 hrs
- Week of surgery: • Instruct in deep breathing maneuvers • Optimize airflow with steroids, bronchodilators • Treat infections • Pulmonary toilet especially if prominent secretions
- Day of surgery: • Schedule late, opportunity to mobilize secretions &toilet • Bronchodilators on call to surgery
- Postoperatively: • Analgesia: especially nerve blocks and epidural narcotics • Early ambulation, incentive spirometry, pulmonary toilet

Preparation for Lung Resection
- pCO2>45 : relative contraindication.
- Pts with airflow obstruction can tolerate resection if
  - Able to climb 2 flights of stairs ≈ MVV > 50% predicted.
  - FEV1 > 2 liters; FEV1/FVC > 50%.
- Radionuclide split perfusion studies: predicted FEV1 > 0.8 postop.
- Pulmonary hypertension: clinical assessment or mean PAP during balloon occlusion of lung to be resected > 30.

Pulmonary Embolism: PIOPED[144]

Comparison of scan category with angiogram findings

Scan category	PE present	PE Absent	PE uncertain	No PAgram	Total
High probability	102	14	1	7	124
Intermediate	105	217	9	33	304
Low probability	39	199	2	74	131
Near-normal	5	50	2	74	131
Total	251	480	24	176	931

Scan category compared with angiogram, sensitivity, specificity

Scan category	Sensitivity %	Specificity %
High probability	41	97
High or intermediate probability	82	52
High, intermediate, or low probability	98	10

---

[143] CV Jackson, "Preoperative pulmonary evaluation," Arch Intern Med 1988;148:2120; Zibrak et al, "Indications for Pulmonary Function Testing," Ann Intern Med 1990;112:763.
[144] "Value of the ventilation/perfusion scan in acute pulmonary embolism: results of the Prospective Investigation of Pulmonary Embolism Diagnosis (PIOPED)," JAMA, 1990;263(20):2753-59.

Pleural Fluid Analysis[145]

Transudates (CHF, nephrosis, cirrhosis, ?PE) EXCLUDED by:
- Pleural/Serum Protein > 0.5
- Pleural LDH > 2/3 upper limit for serum LDH
- Pleural/Serum LDH > 0.6
- Serum albumin - Pleural albumin < 1.2 g/dL[146]

Appearance
- Bloody: "Pleurocrit"/Hematocrit > 0.5 suggests Hemothorax
- Turbid despite centrifugation suggests chlyothorax or pseudochylothorax
- Putrid: suggests empyema
- "Anchovy paste" or "chocolate sauce:" suggests amebiasis

Leukocytes
- WBC's > 10k: pus, pancreatitis, PE, collagen vascular, neoplasm, TB
- Granulocyte predominance: pneumonia, PE, pancreatitis, early TB, abdominal abscess
- Mononuclear predominance: tumor, TB, resolving acute process
- Eosinophil predominance (40% of idiopathic effusions): blood or air in pleural space, asbestos, drugs esp nitrofurantoin or dantrolene, paragonimiasis

Cytology
- Mesothelial cells nonspecific
- Exam may be nondiagnostic for malignancy

Glucose
- < 60 mg/dL: parapneumonic (<40 mg/dL → chest tube), neoplasm, TB, hemothorax, paragonimiasis, Churg-Strauss
- < 30 mg/dL: rheumatoid arthritis

Amylase
- Elevated in: Esophageal perforation, pancreatic disease, malignancy.

LDH
- Nonspecific "indicator of degree of inflammation" and urgency

pH
- < 7: complicated parapneumonic effusion (empyema)
- < 7.20: ? empyema, systemic acidosis, esophageal rupture, rheumatoid arthritis, TB, neoplasm, hemothorax, paragonimiasis

ANA
- > 1:160 or serum level: suggests SLE effusion

Rheumatoid factor
- > 1:320 or serum level: suggests rheumatoid effusion

Adenosine Deaminase
- > 70 IU/L suggests TB; < 40 IU/L makes TB improbable

---

[145] Richard W Light, "Pleural Disease," Disease-A-Month, May 1992.
[146] Roth BJ, et al, "The serum-effusion albumin gradient in the evaluation of pleural effusions," Chest, 1990;98:546-49.

Renal

Metabolic Acidosis

Elevated Anion- Gap
- Renal failure mild: buffered by bone salts
- Accumulation of organic acids
  - Lactic acidosis
  - Ketoacidosis
    - Diabetic: exacerbated by volume contraction
    - Alcoholic: β-OH-butyrate in binge drinkers with anorexia & emesis. Related to reduced insulin secretion. Often with hypoglycemia. Tx glucose & NS.
    - Starvation
  - Ingestion: Salicylates: (1) organic acid. (2). Impair mitochondrial function $\rightarrow$ other acids. (3). Central hyperventilation induced, decreasing bicarb; Methanol (formic acid); Ethylene glycol (glycolic & oxalic acids); Toluene inhalation (glue sniffing); Isoniazid; Iron; Paraldehyde
  - Rhabdomyolysis

Normal Anion Gap (Hyperchloremic)
- Bicarbonate loss
  - GI: diarrhea, ileal drainage, ileal loop (HCO3 exchange for Cl-)
  - Proximal RTA (Type II): Reduced bicarbonate reabsorption set-point. Treat by ECF volume contraction, causing bicarbonate reabsorption
  - Dilutional: decreased sodium & therefore bicarbonate reabsorption
  - Carbonic anhydrase inhibitors (similar to proximal RTA)
  - Primary hyperparathyroidism + hypercalcemia (? mechanism)
- Inadequate bicarbonate reabsorption (see Renal Tubular Acidosis page 84).
  - Distal RTA Type I (adequate H pump, inability to maintain H gradient)
    - Secondary hyperaldosteronism from sodium loss causes hypokalemia
    - Tx with phosphate slates, permit H excretion; or Shohl's + K
  - Type IV RTA (reduced Na absorption, increased K + bicarbonate excretion). (1) Related to drugs (diuretics) (2) Interstitial disease
  - Renal hypoperfusion
- Exogenous acid: Hyperalimentation with inadequate base buffer; Lysine, ammonium, arginine therapy
- Urinary anion gap: index of ammonium excretion; gap positive if intrinsic renal disease (eg RTA), negative if normal or GI bicarbonate loss[147]

Decreased Anion Gap
- Low albumin
- Hyperviscosity syndromes (artifact of flame photometry)
- Multiple myeloma IgG (cationic at pH 7.4)
- Lithium intoxication, hypercalcemia, hypermagnesemia: increased nonsodium cations
- Bromide intoxication (interferes with colorimetry of Cl-)

---

[147] DC Battle *et al*, "The use of the urinary anion gap in the diagnosis of hyperchloremic metabolic acidosis," N Engl J Med 318:594-9, 1988.

Renal Tubular Acidosis[148]

	Distal (Type 1)	Proximal (Type 2)	Type 4
Defect	Inadequate distal acidification	Inadequate proximal HCO_3 reabsorption	Aldosterone deficiency / resistance
Urine pH	> 5.5 (exclude urease-splitting pathogen & extreme hypovolemia)	Variable: > 5.5 if above reabsorptive threshold else < 5.3	≤ 5.5 unless selective aldosterone deficiency
Untreated plasma [HCO_3]	May be < 10 mEq/L	> 12 mEq/L	> 15 mEq/L
Fractional [HCO_3] excretion when plasma [HCO_3] > 20 mEq/L	< 3%	> 15-20%	< 3%
Plasma [K]	Usually ↓-normal; ↑ in Na-reabsorption defect (obstruction, sickle-cell)	Normal or ↓	↑
Urine anion gap (Negative in normals or GI loss)	Positive	Positive	Positive
Diagnosis	Response to $NaHCO_3$ or NH_4Cl	Response to $NaHCO_3$	Plasma aldosterone concentration
Amount $NaHCO_3$ to normalize plasma [HCO_3]	1-3 mEq/kg/d	10-15 mEq/kg/d	1-3 mEq/kg/day or correct hyperkalemia
Other complications	Nephrocalcinosis & lithiasis; osteomalacia uncommon	Children rickets; Adult osteomalacia/penia; calculi rare unless carbonic anhydrase inhibitor	None

NB Type 3 RTA has features of Types I + II.

Lactic Acidosis[149]

Diagnosis
- Exclude CRI, DKA, paraldehyde, salicylates, methanol, ethylene glycol
- Ketoacidosis & LA: altered redox state, β-hydroxybutyrate not detected
- Venous lactate is 50-100% higher than arterial

Type A: Clinicaly apparent hypoperfusion
Pump failure; Anemia/hemorrhage; Hypotension; Sepsis; CO poisoning

Type B: Clinically inapparent hypoperfusion
Common
- Liver disease: In one series seen in fulminant hepatic failure or in chronic disease + acute bleed/sepsis. There were no **marked** alterations in liver function. All had hypoglycemia which, when corrected led to correction of lactic acidosis. No survivors among pts with liver disease & lactic acidosis.

[148] BD Rose and RM Black, "Renal Tubular Acidosis," in <u>Manual of Clinical Problems in Nephrology</u>, Boston: Little, Brown & Company, 1988.
[149] R Green & R Tannen in Kokko JP & Tannen RL (eds) <u>Fluids and Electrolytes</u>, 3/e, Philadelphia: Saunders, 1996.

- Diabetes mellitus: uncertain etiology/setting.
- Hypoglycemia: usually in alcoholics or with enzyme defects.
- Malignant cell production: Usually acute leukemia or lymphoma.
- Seizures, usually transient unless underlying Type A.
- Renal failure.

Drugs & Toxins
- Alcohol: depletion of NAD by ADH; respiratory alkalosis; shock • Fructose & sorbitol (used as insulin-sparing sugars in TPN) • Salicylate-induced hyperventilation • Methanol: Formic & lactic acidosis • Vasopressors
- Nitroprusside: produces cyanide • Cyanide • Isoniazid • Paraldehyde
- Metformin

Hereditary: Gluconeogenesis; Pyruvate oxidation; Mitochondrial myopathies
Short gut syndrome: D-lactate absorbed, not metabolized

Management:
- Underlying condition
- Keep pH > 7.2 (below which cardiac depression begins). Note increased pH causes increased lactate production. Remember V_d HCO_3 = 50% total body weight. Deficit mEq = (Desired HCO_3) × 50% × weight (kg)

Metabolic Alkalosis

Chloride-Responsive ("Contraction"): Urinary Chloride < 10 mEq/L
- GI loss: Emesis, NG suction, villous adenoma, chlorodiarrhea
- Renal loss: Diuretics with restricted Na intake (after drug cleared)
- Posthypercapneic: Increased renal bicarbonate retention
- Bicarbonate load: eg, multiple transfusions (citrate), milk-alkali

Management:
- If volume-contracted: Saline ± KCl
- If volume-overloaded: consider acetazolamide to increase bicarbonate excretion (250-500 mg po/IV q8hrs); consider hemodialysis
- If life-threatening: eg, hepatic encephalopathy, arrhythmias, dig toxicity, alteration in consciousness and if saline is contraindicated:
  - Replace half of H^+-deficit:
    H^+-deficit (mEq/L) = 0.5× wt (kg) × (measured-desired HCO_3 mEq/L).
  - HCl: 0.1N @ 0.2mEq/kg/hr via central line, max 300-500 ml/hr
  - NH_4Cl if no liver/renal dz: 0.1N via peripheral vein, max 300mEq/d

Chloride-Unresponsive: Urinary chloride > 20 mEq/L
- **With hypertension, eg hyperaldosteronism**
  - Low plasma renin
    - Primary aldosteronism or excess mineralocorticoid
    - Glycyrrhizic acid in licorice
  - High plasma renin
    - High plasma cortisol: Cushing syndrome
    - High unilateral renal renin : • Renovascular hypertension • JGA tumor
    - Normal renal vein renin: essential hypertension
  - **Management**: Treat underlying disorder; Restrict Na; Supplement K; Consider K-sparing diuretics (triamterene, amiloride, spironolactone)
- **Without hypertension**
  - **Urinary K < 30 mEq/L**
    - Severe hypokalemia, K < 2 mEq/L • Diuretic/Laxative abuse (urinary K after diuretic worn off)

- **Urinary K > 30 mEq/L**
  - Recent diuretic abuse • Magnesium depletion • Bulimia with vomiting
  - Barrter syndrome (impaired chloride resorption in loop of Henle or distal tubule, typically woman < 30 years): tx NSAIDS

Hyponatremia

Isoosmolar (Pseudohyponatremia, artifact of flame photometry, not of ion-specific electrodes). Correction:
  - % Serum H_2O = 99 - 1.03×(Lipid g/dL) - 0.73×(Protein g/dL)
  - Na corrected = Na measured × 93/(% serum H_2O)
  - Protein > 10 g/dL • Profound hyperlipidemia

Hyperosmolar (> 285 mOsm/L)
  - Mannitol infusions
  - Hyperglycemia (Na decreased 1.6mM for each 100mg/dL Glucose)

Hypoosmolar (< 280 mOsm/L)
  - Volume-contracted
    - Renal losses (U_{Na}>20mM): • Diuretic excess & osmotic diuresis
      • Mineralocorticoid deficiency • Partial obstruction • Salt-losing nephropathy
      • Bicarbonaturia: (RTA, Metabolic acidosis; Ketonuria)
    - Extrarenal loss: (U_{Na}<10mM): • Vomiting • Diarrhea • "Third-spacing," eg pancreatitis
  - Volume-overloaded
    - Congestive heart failure; Cirrhosis; Nephrotic syndrome (U_{Na}<10mM)
    - Impaired water excretion: acute & chronic renal failure (U_{Na}>20mM)
  - Euvolemic
    - U_{Na} > 20mM: • Hypothyroidism • Adrenal insufficiency • SIADH • Renal failure
    - Psychogenic polydipsia (U_{Na} < 10 mM, U_{osm}<80mOsm/L)

Management:
• Sodium deficit = 0.6 × body wt (kg) × {125 - [Serum Na]} (in mmol)
• Acute symptomatic hyponatremia (onset 1-3 days):
Replace 1-2mEq/L/hr with 0.9 or 3.0% NaCl Caution: Excessively-rapid
correction of hyponatremia may cause central pontine myelinolysis.
• Chronic hyponatremia: Replace 0.5 mEq/L/hr with 0.9% NaCl

Hypernatremia[150]

Dehydration

Excess mineralocorticoids
  • Hyperaldosteronism • Cushing sydnrome • Congenital adrenal hyperplasia

Central diabetes insipidus
  • Idiopathic: Familial; Sporadic • Trauma: Basal skull fracture; surgical manipulation of pituitary fossa • Vascular: Aneurysms; Thrombosis; Sheehan's syndrome • Tumor: Neoplasm, Sarcoidosis, Histiocytosis X • Postencephalitic; postmeningitic, Lyme Borreliosis • Guillain Barré syndrome

Nephrogenic diabetes insipidus
  • Idiopathic/congenital • Renal disease: Nonoliguric ATN; cystic disease; postobstructive; amyloid; myeloma; sickle cell disease; Sjögren syndrome • Electrolytes: Hypercalcemia; severe hypokalemia • Osmotic diuresis: tube feeds; glucose; mannitol; glycerol; urea • Drugs: demeclocycline; lithium; amphotericin; colchicine; methoxyflurane

---

[150] Kassirer, Hricik, Cohen, Repairing Body Fluids, Philadelphia: Saunders, 1989.

Management:

Most pts have accompanying sodium deficit; give NS if volume-depleted.
Mortality exceeds 60% when Na>160 for more than 48hrs
Water deficit = ((Na / 140) - 1) × TBW;   TBW=0.6×weight.
Correct deficit over 48-72 hrs ~ 0.5-1.0 mM/hr.
Central DI: Desmopressin 10-20μg nasal qd-bid.

Potassium

Hypokalemia   Note: decrease in K 4.0→3.0 ≅ 300 mmol total body loss
- Exogenous
  - <u>Inadequate intake</u> • <u>GI loss</u>: vomiting, diarrhea, laxatives, urinary diversion, villous adenoma • <u>Renal loss</u>: • Diuretics • Alkalosis, mineralocorticoid excess, licorice, hyperreninemia (tumors, renovascular HTN, Bartter's) • Renal tubular acidosis, distal and proximal • Leukemias (lysozymuria) • <u>Polyanionic drugs</u>, eg carbenicillin • <u>Hypomagnesemia</u>
- Endogenous
  - Excessive insulin, eg, parenteral glucose infusion • β-2 adrenergic agonists • Periodic paralysis: familial or thyrotoxic (more common in Asians) • Correction of megaloblastic anemia (cellular incorporation)

Management:

- For K<2.0 accompanied by paralysis, arrhythmia, rhabdomyolysis: KCl 20-40 mEq/hr IV with continuous ECG monitoring.
- Otherwise, KCl 20-40 mEq po q 2-24hr, check serum K after each dose. May also give 10-20mEq KCl/hr IV as 20-40 mEq/L.
- Reverse underlying cause (eg diuretic).
- Treat associated electrolyte disorders (eg reverse ↓ Mg, contraction alkalosis).

Hyperkalemia
- Factitious: hemolysis; thrombocytosis or leukocytosis (**plasma** K normal).
- Exogenous: excessive intake; tissue destruction; K-sparing diuretics
  Rarely seen in absence of • Renal insufficiency or tubulointerstitial disease
  • Tubular unresponsivenes to **aldosterone** (eg sickle cell, SLE, diabetes, obstruction, cyclosporine) • Drug: ACE inhibitor, NSAID, heparin (esp RTA-4), K-sparing diuretic
- Endogenous
  - Acidosis (mineral not organic acids) • Insulin-deficiency, eg DKA • Hyperosmolarity drives K out of cells • β-adrenergic agonists • Digitalis toxicity (severe) inhibits Na-K-ATPase • Succinylcholine, esp with neuromuscular dz, neuropathy (eg DM)

Urgent management (cardiac repolarization abnormalities)
- Temporize:
  - IV Calcium gluconate 1 Amp ("cardioprotective")
  - Insulin 10-20 units IV
  - Dextrose 50% 1 amp IV
  - Bicarbonate 1 amp IV
  - ? aerosolized albuterol
- Remove body potassium definitively
  - Sodium polystyrene sulfonate (kayexalate) po or enema
  - Dialysis if renal failure

Calcium[151]

Hypercalcemia
- Parathyroid-related ($\uparrow$ 1,25(OH)$_2$D; $\uparrow$ PTH): 1° hyperparathyroidism: solidary adenoma; MEN-I,IIa; Lithium; Familial hypocalciuric $\uparrow$ Ca
- Malignancy ($\downarrow$ 1,25(OH)$_2$D; $\downarrow$ PTH):
  Bone metastases(eg breast); humorally-mediated hypercalcemia (eg lung, kidney); Hematologic malignancy (eg multiple myeloma, lymphoma, leukemia)
- Vitamin-D-related: Vitamin D intoxication; Elevated 1,25(OH)$_2$-D: granulomatous diseases; Idiopathic hypercalcemia of infancy
- High bone turnover: Hyperthyroidism; Immobilization; Thiazides; Vitamin A intoxication
- Renal failure: Secondary hyperparathyroidism; Aluminum intoxication; Milk-alkali syndrome

Management:
- Hydration ± diuretics (eg 4-6 L NS IV + furosemide q 1-2h + K 60 mEq/d + Mg 60 mmol/d)
- Plicamycin (mithramycin) 25 μg/kg IV over 4 hrs × 1
- Oral phosphorus (250 mg P q 6h until P > 3 mg/dL)
- Bisphosphonates (eg pamidronate 60-90 mg IV over 24hr)
- Glucocorticoids (eg prednisone 20-60 mg/d; esp hematologic malignancies, granulomatous disease, vitamin D intoxication)
- Dialysis in acute renal failure
- Calcitonin (adjunct in bone reabs & immobilization; 2-8U/kg SQ q 4h)
- IV phosphate (in severe $\uparrow$Ca and dialysis/plicamycin contraindicated; 1500 mg P q 12h until [P]>2mmol/L; can cause fatal $\downarrow$ Ca & metastatic calcification)
- Gallium nitrate 200mg/m^{2}BSA in 1L over 24° × 5d

Hypocalcemia
- PTH absent: hereditary/acquired hypoparathyroidism; hypomagnesemia
- PTH ineffective
- Chronic renal failure
- Inadequate active vitamin D: Inadequate dietary intake or sunlight; Defective metabolism: Anticonvulsant drugs; Vitamin-D-dependent rickets type I
- Ineffective active vitamin D: (1) Intestinal malabsorption; (2) Vitamin-D-dependent rickets type II
- Pseudohypoparathyroidism
- PTH overwhelmed
- Severe, acute hyperphosphatemia: tumor lysis, acute renal failure; rhabdomyolysis
- Osteitis fibrosa after parathyroidectomy ("hungry bone syndrome")

---

[151] JP Bilezikian, "Management of acute hypercalcemia," N Engl J Med 1992; 326(18):1196. JT Potts, "Diseases of the parathyroid gland and other hyper- and hypo-calcemic disorders," in Isselbacher KJ et al (eds), Harrison's Principles of Internal Medicine, 13/e, NY: McGraw-Hill, 1994, pp 2151-2171.

Diuretic Resistance[152]

Normal renal sodium handling

(1) Normal FENa > 1%; (2) Proximal tubule reabsobs 2/3 filtered Na mostly via electroneutral Na-H exchange (3) Loop of Henle reabsorbs ¼ filtered Na. Thin descending and ascending limb absorption mostly via passive exchange of Na,K,2Cl across lumen; (4) Distal tubule reabsorbs 5-10% filtered Na, probably via directly coupled NaCl pathway without K; (5) Collecting duct reabsorbs 3% filtered NaCl, via electrogenic pathways.

How diuretics work

- Carbonic anhydrase inhibitors at proximal tubule: ↓ H^+ available for exchange with Na. **Weak** due to compensatory ↑ distal Na absorption.
- Loop diuretics: inhibit Na-K-2Cl exchange at luminal surface of thick ascending limb; blocks most NaCl transport. No effect on distal tubule. **Potent** because distal Na delivery exceeds distal reabsorptive capacity.
- Thiazides: act on distal convoluted tubule, from the luminal surface, inhibits coupled NaCl movement across luminal membrane.
- Collecting duct: Na-channel blockers: amiloride & triamterene block Na uptake and ↓ lumen negative voltage, thereby sparing K secretion. Minimal additional effect at proximal tubule.
- Collecting duct: Aldosterone antagonist spironolactone.

Renal Adaptation to Diuretics

- Compensatory distal reabsoption of increased distal sodium delivery. Blunts effect of proximal tubule. but not loop. and distal. diuretics.
- Compensatory "postdiuretic" NaCl retention, related to ↓ ECF volume, ↑ renal nerve activity, circulating aldosterone. **Must restrict dietary Na!**
- ECF depletion reduces filtered NaCl available for tubular reabsoption.
- Distal tubule hypertrophy/hyperfunction in chronic ↑ distal NaCl delivery.

Elements of Diuretic Resistance

- Patient noncompliance: not taking drug; high salt intake
- ↓ drug delivery to tubular lumen: (1) ↓ bioavailability, eg bowel edema from CHF; (2) Blocked of organic acid/base secretion: NSAIDS, uremic toxins, probenecid; (3) Protein binding in tubule: nephrotic syndrome;
- Hemodynamic ↓ GFR: (1) Excessive afterload ↓ or BP ↓; (2) Hypoxemia
- ↑ NaCl reabsoption: 1º: cirrhosis, CHF; 2º:chronic diuretic adaptation

Overcoming Diuretic resistance

- 24hr urine Na to assess compliance: Reduce NaCl intake if > 100mmol/d

---

[152]DH Ellison "The physiologic basis of diuretic synergism: its role in treating diuretic resistance, " Ann Intern Med 1991;114(10):886-894.

Rheumatology

ARA Criteria for SLE classification[153]

Four or more of the following criteria
- **Malar rash**: fixed erythema, flat or raised, over malar eminences, tending to spare the nasolabial folds
- **Discoid rash**: erythematous raised patches with adherent keratotic scaling and follicular plugging; atrophic scarring may occur in older lesions
- **Photosensitivity**: Skin rash as a result of unusual reaction to sunlight, by patient history or physician observation
- **Oral ulcers**: Oral or nasolabial ulceration, usually painless, seen by MD
- **Arthritis**: nonerosive arthritis involving two or more peripheral joints, characterized by tenderness, swelling, or effusion
- Serositis:
  - **Pleuritis**: convincing history of pleuritic pain or rub heard by a physician or evidence of pleural effusion, **or**
  - **Pericarditis**: by ECG or rub or evidence of pericardial effusion
- Renal disorder:
  - Persistent **proteinuria** > 0.5 grams per day or greater than 3+, **or**
  - Cellular **casts**: may be RBC, hemoglobin, granular, tubular, or mixed **or**
- Neurologic disorder
  - **Seizures** or **Psychosis**: in absence of offending drugs or known metabolic derangement, eg uremia, ketoacidosis, or electrolyte imbalance
- Hematologic disorder:
  - **Hemolytic anemia**, with reticulocytosis, **or** **Leukopenia**, < 4,000 total on two or more occasions, **or** **Lymphopenia** < 1,500 on two or more occasions, **or** **Thrombocytopenia** < 100,000 in absence of offending drugs
- Immunologic disorder
  - Positive **LE cell preparation**, **or** **Anti-ds-DNA** antibody, **or** **Anti-Sm** antibody, **or** **False-positive** nontreponemal test for **syphilis** (eg VDRL, RPR) > 6 months with negative treponemal test for syphilis (eg FTA, MHATP)
- **Antinuclear antibody**: without drugs typical of "drug-induced" lupus syndrome

ARA Criteria: Rheumatoid Arthritis[154]

Four of the following   * For 6 weeks or longer
- **Morning stiffness*** In and around the joints, lasting at least one hour
- **Arthritis of three or more joint areas***
  Simultaneous soft tissue swelling or fluid observed by an MD, > 2 joint areas
- **Arthritis of hand joints*** At least one area swollen in a wrist, MCP, or PIP joint
- **Symmetric arthritis*** Simultaneous involvement of same joint areas on both sides of the body
- **Rheumatoid nodules** Subcutaneous nodules observed by an MD
- **Serum rheumatoid factor:** False-positive test in 5% of normals (by definition)
- **Radiographic changes:** Erosions or unequivocal bony decalcification localized in or most marked adjacent to involved hand & wrist joints

---

[153] Adapted from EM Tan et al, "The 1982 revised criteria for the classification of systemic lupus erythematosus (SLE), Arthritis Rheum 25:1271-7, 1982.
[154] FC Arnett, et al, "American Rheumatism Association 1987 revised criteria for the classification of rheumatoid arthritis," Arthritis Rheum, 31:315-24, 1988.

Arthritis & Fever[155]

Causes

Diagnosis	Confirm
Infectious arthritis	
Septic arthritis	Culture
Bacterial endocarditis	Blood Cx
Lyme disease	Serology
Mycobacteria/fungi	Culture, Bx
Viral arthritis	Serology
Postinfectious/reactive	
Enteric	Cx/serology
Reiter's (urogenital)	Culture
Rheumatic fever	Clinical
Inflammatory bowel	Clinical
Systemic rheumatic dz	
Systemic vasculitis	Biopsy/angio
SLE	Serology
Rheumatoid arthritis	Clinical
Still's disease	Clinical
Crystal-arthritis	
Gout / pseudogout	Polarized
Other diseases	
Familial Med. Fever	Clinical
Cancers	Biopsy
Sarcoidosis	Biopsy
Mucocutaneous dz	
Dermatomyositis	
Behçet disease	
Henoch-Schöenlein	
Kawasaki disease	
Erythema nodosum	
Erythema multiforme	
Pyoderma gangr'sum	
Pustular psoriasis	

> **Prompt arthrocentesis essential!**
> Gram stain 50-75% sensitive;
> Culture >90% sensitive
> for diagnosis of septic arthritis

Distinguishing features

Symptom/Sign	Possible diagnosis
T > 40ºC	Still's disease; SLE
	Bacterial arthritis
Antecedent fever	Viral; Lyme
	Reactive; Still's dz
	Bacterial endocarditis
Migratory arthritis	Rheumatic fever
	Neisseria spp.
	Viral arthritis; SLE
	Acute leukemia
	Whipple's disease
Effusion >> Pain	Tuberculous arthritis
	Bacterial endocarditis
	Inflammatory bowel
	Giant-cell arteritis
	Lyme disease
Pain >> effusion	Rheumatic fever
	Familial Mediterran. Fever
	Acute leukemia
	AIDS
(+) Rheumatoid factor	Rheumatoid arthritis
	Viral arthritis
	Tuberculous arthritis
	Bacterialendocarditis
	Sarcoidosis; SLE
	Systemic vasculitis
Morning stiffness	Rheumatoid arthritis
	Polymyalgia rheum.
	Still's disease
	Some viral/reactive
Symmetric small-joint synovitis	Rheumatoid arthritis
	SLE
	Viral arthritis
WBC > 15k/mm³	Bacterial arthritis
	Bacterial endocarditis
	Still's disease
	Systemic vasculitis
	Acute leukemia
Leukopenia	SLE; Viral arthritis
Episodic recurrences	Crystal-induced
	Inflammatory bowel
	Lyme; Whipple
	Familial Med. Fever
	Still's disease; SLE

---

155 RS Pinals, "Polyarthritis and fever," N Engl J Med, 1994; 330(11):769. Reprinted with permission of *The New England Journal of Medicine*, Copyright 1994, Massachusetts Medical Society.

Autoantibodies[156]

Antibody	Sensitivity	Known antigen	Comment
ANA	SLE 95%, many other CTD	Multiple nuclear & cytoplasmic Ab's	Repeated (-) makes SLE unlikely. Human lines more sensitive than murine. Detects multiple Ab's. False(+) usually low-titer, elderly, homogeneous pattern.
α-ssDNA	SLE 30-70%; CAH	DNA	Associated with clinical **activity** and **nephritis**. dsDNA specific; ssDNA not.
α-Sm	SLE<30%	Protein & 6sRNA	Specific for SLE but insensitive
α-RNP	SLE 40%, MCTD, other CTD	U1-RNP	Risk for SLE **nephritis** low if α-DNA (-). High titer (>1:10k) in polymyositis, scleroderma, SLE, MCTD.
α-Ro (SSA)	SS 75%; SLE 25-30%; other CTD esp. with SS	Protein-Y1-Y5 RNA complex	Associated with SLE **nephritis**. Sjogren's, DR3 haplotype, subacute cutaneous LE (85%), inherited complement defic'y, ANA(-) SLE, elderly or neonates, CHB (>85%).
α-La (SSB)	SS 40%; SLE 10%; other CTD	Phosphoprotein + RNA pol III transcripts	Always associated with α-Ra. Low risk of **nephritis** in SLE. Congenital CHB
α-Histone	Drug SLE>90% other SLE>50%		Nonspecific by sensitive for drug-induced SLE
α-Cardiolipin	50%		Venous & arterial thrombosis, ↓ Plt, spontaneous Ab, ↑ PTT, false-(+) VDRL.
α-RBC	60%		Infrequent hemolysis.
α-Platelet	—		Low platelets
α-Lymphocyte	70%		Leukopenia & ↓ T cell fxn.
α-Neuronal	60%		↑ CSF IgG: diffuse CNS SLE.
α-Centromere	CREST>80%		Limited scleroderma (CREST)
α-SCL-70	66%	Topoisomerase-I	Diffuse scleroderma (PSS) only.
α-Jo-1	25%	Histidyl-tRNA synthetase	Dermato/Myositis (25%), overlap syndromes incl pulm fibrosis
c-ANCA[157]	active WG>90%, WG 10%	PR3 protease	Wegener granulomatosis
p-ANCA		Myeloperoxidase	Crescentic GN,IBD,RA,liver

Abbreviations: α=anti; Ab=antibody, abortion; ANA=antinuclear antibody; CAH=chronic active hepatitis; CHB=complete heart block; CREST=calcinosis, Raynaud, esophageal dysmotility, sclerodactyly, telangiectasia; CTD=connective tissue disease; dsDNA=double-stranded DNA; GN=glomerulonephritis; IBD=inflammatory bowel disease; MCTD=Mixed CTD; PSS=Progressive systemic sclerosis; SLE=systemic lupus erythematosus; SS=Sjögren syndrome; ssDNA=single stranded DNA; WG=Wegener granulomatosis

[156] Moder KG, "Use and interpretation of rheumatologic tests: a guide for clinicians," Mayo Clin Proc, 1996;71(4):391-6. JD Wilson et al (eds), Harrison's Principles of Internal Medicine 12/e 1991,NY:McGraw-Hill
[157] C Kallenberg et al, "ANCA," Am J Med, 1992; 93:675.

Synovial Fluid Analysis

Patterns

	Normal	Inflammatory	Non-Inflammatory	Infectious	Hemorrhagic
Appearance	Clear	Clear yellow	Cloudy, Yellow	Opaque, purulent	Opaque, red
Viscosity	High	High	Low	Low	Variable
WBC/mm^3	<200	<3000	2000-75,000	50k-300k	Variable
PMNs	<25%	<25%	50-100%	75-100%	Variable
Glucose ratio joint/serum	0.9-1.0	0.9-1.0	0.4-0.9	<0.5	0.9-1.0

Crystals • Negatively birefringent (yellow when ||, blue when ⊥ to polarized axis): urate: thin spindly (gout), betamethasone, calcium oxalate & lithium heparin
• Positively birefringent (yellow-paraellel, blue-perpendicular); calcium pyrophosphate (pseudogout) short rhomboid crystals weakly (+)

Noninflammatory pattern • Degenerative joint disease • Trauma • Chronic or subsiding crystal synovitis • Avascular necrosis • SLE, polyarteritis • Acute rheumatic fever • Endocrine arthropathy

Inflammatory pattern • Crystal synovitis • Rheumatoid arthritis; • Spondyloarthropathy; • Reactive arthritis; • Juvenile RA • Acute rheumatic fever • Sarcoidosis • Viral arthritis

Septic pattern: Gram stain/culture yield high for GPCs/GNRs not GC
• Bacterial, fungal, TB infection • Rheumatoid arthritis • Crystal synovitis

Hemorrhagic pattern: • Trauma, fracture, Charcot joint, sickle-cell disease
• Coagulopathy: hemophilia, warfarin, thrombocytopenia • Tumor • Pigmented villonodular synovitis

Groovy Drugs

Acetylcysteine[158]

Action: Repletes hepatic reducing capacity in acetaminophen overdose. May have role in fulminant hepatic failure & in overcoming nitrate tachyphylaxis.

PO: 140 mg/kg then 70 mg/kg q4hr x 17 doses. Dilute to 5% in cola or juice. Repeat dose if patient vomits.

IV: 140 mg/kg (in 200 mL D5W over 15 min), then 50mg/kg (in 500mL D5W over 4 hr), then 100mg/kg (in 100mL D5W over 16 hr). Not FDA-approved.

Side-effects: N/V, stomatitis, drowsiness, rash, bronchospasm, odor.

Interactions: Activated charcoal prevents oral absorption; stagger other medications by 1-2 hours.

Adenosine[159] (Adenocard)

Action: Slows AV node conduction. Locally-acting coronary vasodilator. T½ <10 seconds, metabolized by RBCs. Use to diagnose wide-complex tachycardias, and to interrupt reentrant tachycardias involving AV node. Efficacy comparable to verapamil with shorter T½. Also used as coronary vasodilator (ie perfusion imaging, rotational atherectomy).

IV: 6mg IV RAPID PUSH & FLUSH within 3 seconds, repeat 12mg after one minute and may repeat 12-18 mg if no response. Give via central venous line if possible. Double dose for methylxanthines; halve for disopyramide. Myocardial perfusion imaging: 175 mcg/kg/min × 6 min.

Warnings: Avoid in WPW or irregular wide-complex rhythms (may cause anterograde bypass tract conduction in WPW/a-fib). Causes transient 1-3rd degree heart block or asystole. May cause bronchospasm.

Interactions: Competitively antagonized by methylxanthines. Potentiated by dipyridamole (nucleoside transport inhibitor) & carbamazepine, reported to cause high-grade AV block.

Pregnancy: Class C; no fetal effects anticipated.

Side-effects: Transient: flushing, lightheaded, dyspnea, nausea, angina.

Amiodarone IV[160] (Cordarone)

Action: Complex antiarrhythmic with sodium, potassium, calcium, and beta-blocking activity. Used IV in critically ill pts with sustained or recurrent life-threatening ventricular arrhythmia refractory to lidocaine, procainamide, ± bretylium. Compared to bretylium, ↓ hypotension & comparable efficacy. Unlike oral formulation, prolongs AV nodal refractoriness without short-term effect on SA node, intraventricular conduction, or QT interval.

Kinetics: Rapid redistribution → 10% peak concentration 30-45 min after infusion. Rapid effect attributed to high serum concentration. T½ probably exceeds 30d.

IV: Best administered through central vein. Load 150 mg (in 100mL D5W) over 10

[158] MJ Smilkstein, et al, "Efficacy of oral n-acetylcysteine in the treatment of acetaminophen overdose," N Engl J Med 319:1557, 1988; PM Harrison, et al, "Improvement by acetylcysteine of hemodynamics and oxygen transport in fulminant hepatic failure," N Engl J Med, 324:1852, 1991.

[159] JP DiMarco, et al, "Adenosine for paroxysmal supraventricular tachycardia: dose ranging and comparison with verapamil," Ann Intern Med 113(2):104-10, 1990.

[160] GV Nacarelli, S Jalal, "Intravenous amiodarone: another option in the acute management of sustained ventricular tachyarrhthmias," Circulation 1995; 92:3154-55; PR Kowel et al, "Randomized, double-blind comparison of intravenous amiodarone and bretylium in the treatment of patients with recurrent, hemodynamically destabilizing ventricular tachycardia or fibrillation, Circulation 1995; 92:3255-63; MM Scheinman et al, "Dose-ranging study of intravenous amiodarone in patients with life-threatening ventricular tachyarrhythmias," Circulation 1995; 92:3264-72. JH Levine et al "Intravenous amiodarone for recurrent sustained hypotensive ventricular tachyarrhythmias," J Am Coll Cardiol 1996;27:67-75.

min then 900 mg in 500mL D5W @ 1 mg/min x 6 hr then 0.5 mg/min x 18 hr. **Breakthrough** events: bolus 150mg/100mL over 10 min. **Maintenance** 0.5 mg/min.

Rapid-load oral[161]: 400 mg po then 200 mg po q 2 hr x 12-48 hr, as tolerated.
Renal failure, liver failure: No dose-adjustment thought warranted.
Side effects: Hypotension, CHF, Torsades, nodal rhythm, phlebitis, nausea, confusion, biochemical hepatitis, thrombocytopenia, fever.
Interactions: Precipitates with aminophylline, heparin, acetic acid or acetate, mezlocillin, cefamandole, cefazolin.

Aminoglycosides

Divided dosing: Based on lean body weight.

Drug	Load	Total daily	Divided	Peak / Trough (µg/mL)
Gentamicin Tobramycin Netilmicin	1.5-2 mg/kg	3-5 mg/kg	q 8 hr	4-6 / 1-2
Amikacin	7.5-15 mg/kg	15 mg/kg	q 12 hr	20-35 / < 5
Streptomycin	7.5-15 mg/kg	15mg/kg (<2g/d)	q 12 hr	20-30 / < 5

Once-daily dosing[162] Efficacy probably comparable to divided dosing, but nephrotoxicity and ototoxicity are reduced. Gentamicin, tobramycin, or netilmicin 3-6 mg/kg IV qd, check levels after 48hrs, otherwise q week. Restrict to patients with normal renal function. Infuse over 60 min to avoid neuromuscular blockade.
Levels: Draw peak/trough specimens 30 min before/after dose infused. Adjust *dosage* based on peak levels, *intervals* based on trough levels.
Renal failure: Anuric: Supplement: Hemodialysis: 2/3 normal dose after each hemodialysis (½ normal dose for streptomycin). CAPD/CAVH: 3-4 mg/L/d gent/netil/tobra; 15-20 mg/L/d amikacin; 20-40 mg/L/d streptomycin.
Oliguric: Adjust dose according to estimated creatinine clearance:

$$CL_{cr} \, (ml/min) = \frac{140 - Age \, (yrs)}{Serum \, Creatinine \, (mg/dL) \times 72} \times Weight \, (kg) \, (x \, 0.85 \, If \, Woman)$$

Give half of loading dose each half-life interval, or follow table[163]:

CLcr (mL/min)	Half-life (hr)	Dose q 8 hr	Dose q 12 hr	Dose q 24 hr
90	3.1	84%	—	—
80	3.4	80%	91%	—
70	3.9	76%	88%	—
60	4.5	71%	84%	—
50	5.3	65%	79%	—
40	6.5	57%	72%	92%
30	8.4	48%	63%	86%
25	9.9	43%	57%	81%
20	11.9	—	—	75%
17	13.6	—	—	70%
15	15.1	—	—	67%
10	20.4	—	—	56%
<10	25-70	—	—	20%

Adverse Reactions: Nephrotoxicity, especially in volume-depletion, liver disease, prolonged therapy, elderly, concurrent nephrotoxic drugs. High-frequency

[161] BB Massie, personal communication, October 1995; Regimen designed to limit GI intolerance
[162] JM Prins et al, "Once versus thrice daily gentamicin in patients with serious infections," Lancet 1993; 341:335; JM Barza et al, "Single or multiple daily doses of aminoglycosides: a meta-analysis," BMJ 1996;312:338-345; R Hatala, et al, "Once-daily aminoglycoside dosing in immunocompetent adults: a meta-analysis," Ann Intern Med 1996; 124:717-7125.
[163] FA Sarubbi and JH Hull, "Amikacin serum concentrations: prediction of levels and dosage guidelines," Ann Intern Med, 1978;89:612-8.

ototoxicity irreversible, not assessable without special audiologic testing. Neuromuscular blockade especially with intraperitoneal or rapid IV infusion, or in myasthenia gravis; reverse with IV calcium.

Aminophylline

<u>Action:</u> Phosphodiesterase inhibitor and nonspecific adenosine antagonist. Used as bronchodilator in acute and chronic bronchospasm, to reverse intravenous dipyridamole, and as weak diuretic. May reduce contrast nephropathy[164]. Therapeutic window is narrow and efficacy therefore controversial[165].

<u>Levels</u> 10-20 µg/dL therapeutic; > 20 µg/dL risk seizure, arrhythmia. Measure levels 30 min after IV load; 4-8hrs after maintenance infusion.

<u>IV:</u> **Loading dose:** 5.5mg/kg IV over 20min if not already using aminophylline. If already on methylxanthines, each 0.5mg/kg increases theophylline levels by 1µ /mL; if levels unavailable, empiric load 2.5mg/kg.

Maintenance	1st 12 hours	Followed by:
Smokers	1mg/kg/hr	0.8mg/kg/hr
Nonsmokers	0.7mg/kg/hr	0.5mg/kg/hr
Geriatric & cor pulmonale	0.6mg/kg/hr	0.3mg/kg/hr
CHF & Liver dz	0.5mg/kg/hr	0.1-0.2mg/kg/hr

<u>PO:</u> Theophylline=0.85×Aminophylline. **Load:** 6mg/kg theophylline for naive pts.

Maintenance	After load	Followed by:
Smokers	3mg/kg q4x3	q6
Nonsmokers	3mg/kg q4x2	q8
Geriatric & cor pulmonale	2mg/kg q4x2	q8
CHF & Liver dz	2mg/kg q8x2	1-2mg/kg q12

Peak levels 3-12hr (sustained), 1-2hr (normal). Measure 3d after Δ.

<u>Renal failure:</u> No adjustment. Supplement ½ dose after hemodialysis.

<u>Interactions & Elimination:</u> half-time 8.7hrs healthy nonsmoker, 4.4 hrs in smokers. **Shortened** by phenytoin, barbiturates, tobacco (4.4hrs), marijuana, childhood (4hrs). **Lengthened** by CHF or cirrhosis (20-30hrs), neonates, erythromycin, cimetidine, propranolol, allopurinol.

<u>Pregnancy:</u> Neonates sometimes have signs of theophylline toxicity. Nursing infants may receive up to 10% maternal dose.

Amrinone (Inocor)

<u>Action:</u> Inotrope-vasodilator. Additive to digoxin and catecholamines; potent direct systemic, pulmonary, coronary vasodilator. Reportedly little Δ in M$_v$O$_2$. Resembles dobutamine hemodynamically with less tachyphylaxis. Increases infarct size in dogs. Used acutely in CHF refractory to diuretics, afterload reduction.

<u>Kinetics:</u> Hepatic/renal clearance. T½ 2.6-8.3 h.

<u>IV:</u> **Bolus** 0.75 mg/kg over 2-3 min then 5-10µg/kg/min (max 10mg/kg/day). May **rebolus** 0.75 mg/kg 30 min after starting therapy. <u>Mix:</u> Add 300mg (60mL) to 60mL NS (not D5) for 2500µg/mL. May coinfuse with dextrose.

<u>Renal failure:</u> Give 50-75% dose for GFR<10mL/min.

<u>Side Effects:</u> Vasodilation/hypotension (dose-related) especially if hypovolemic, thrombocytopenia (1-2%, dose-related), increased AV conduction with increased

[164] Katholi RE, et al, "Nephrotoxicity from contrast media: attenuation with theophylline," Radiology, 1995;195(1):17-22.

[165] Huang D, et al, "Does aminophylline benefit adults admitted to the hospital for an acute exacerbation of asthma?" Ann Intern Med, 1993;119(12):1155-60. Wrenn K, et al, "Aminophylline therapy for acute bronchospastic disease in the emergency room," Ann Intern Med, 1991;115(4):241-7. Lam A; Newhouse MT, "Management of asthma and chronic airflow limitation. Are methylxanthines obsolete?" Chest, 1990;98(1):44-52. Self TH, et al, "Inhaled albuterol and oral prednisone therapy in hospitalized adult asthmatics. Does aminophylline add any benefit?" Chest, 1990;98(6):1317-21. Murata GH, et al, "Aminophylline in the outpatient management of decompensated chronic obstructive pulmonary disease," Chest, 1990; 98(6):1346-50.

v-response in atrial fib; idiosyncratic hepatotoxicity, N/V/abd discomfort. Caution: A-fib, hypotension, hypertrophic cardiomyopathy.

Anticholinesterases[166]

Neostigmine, Physostigmine, Pyridostigmine. See edrophonium on page 103.

Action: Reversible anticholinesterase inhibitors, ↑ ACh concentration by blocking degradation. Restore muscle contraction. ↓ intraocular pressure. Action resembles organophosphates (irreversible anticholinesterases).

Indications: (1) Antagonize nondepolarizing neuromuscular blockers. (2) myasthenia gravis. (3) Anticholinergic neurotoxicity: CNS (delirium, hallucinations, seizure, hyperactivity) and peripheral (tachycardia, fever, mydriasis, vasodilation, urinary retention, reduced GI motility, reduced upper respiratory secretions). Culprit drugs include atropine, belladonna alkaloids, TCAs, phenothiazines, neuromuscular blockers, antihistamines. (4) GI ileus & bladder atony. (5) Open-angle glaucoma.

Warning: Reversing neuromuscular blockade: co-administer atropine or glycopyrrolate to avoid muscarinic effects eg bradycardia/asystole, salivation, etc. Care in setting of asthma, DM, obstructed viscus.

Side effects: Cholinergic crisis. Bradycardia, seizures, esp. given too-rapidly. Bronchospasm. Excessive salivation, emesis, urination, defecation.

Interactions: Prolong effects of succinylcholine. Antagonized by Class 1a anti-arrhythmics, magnesium, corticosteroids. Causes severe hypotension used with ganglionic blockers.

Physostigmine
Indication: Anticholinergic drug toxicity. Tertiary amine crosses blood-brain barrier unlike neostigmine.
Kinetics: Onset 1-5 min. Duration 45-90 min.
IV: 2mg (0.2mg/kg pediatric) IV < 1mg/min. Repeat prn.

Pyridostigmine
Indication: Antagonize nondepolarizing neuromuscular blockade, myasthenia gravis (oral dosing).
Kinetics: Onset 2-5 min IV, duration 2-3 hr. T½ 1.5-2hrs (ESRD 6hr).
IV: 10-30 mg after atropine 0.6-1.2 mg or with glycopyrrolate 7 µg/kg.
Renal failure: GFR>50: 50%; GFR 10-50: 35%; GFR<10: 20% dose.

Neostigmine
Indication: Antagonize nondepolarizing neuromuscular blocker, ileus, myasthenia gravis.
Kinetics: Onset 4-8 min IV, duration 2-4 hrs. T½ 1.3 hrs (ESRD 3hr).
IV: 0.5-2.5 mg preceded by atropine 0.6-1.2 mg IV or with glycopyrrolate 7 µg/kg. For ileus: 0.25-1.0 mg SQ/IM q 4-6 hrs.
Renal failure: GFR 10-50: 50%; GFR<10: 25% dose.

Atracurium
See "Neuromuscular blockers" on page 111.

Atropine

Action: Muscarinic acetylcholine receptor antagonist. Blocks vagal influence on SA and AV nodes reversing functional bradycardia & AV block. Inhaled bronchodilator in severe bronchospasm, significant systemic absorption (unlike ipratropium). Reduces oropharyngeal secretions for endotracheal intubation. Also used to counteract organophosphate & anticholinesterase drugs/toxicity.
Kinetics: Hepatic metabolism. Onset 1-2 min; T½ 2 hr initially then 13hrs.
IV: **Bradycardia:** 0.5-1.0 mg q 5 min max 0.04mg/kg (2 mg). May be administered via endotracheal tube. **Anticholinesterase poisoning:** 2mg IV/IM q 20 min until muscarinic symptoms disappear, max 6 mg/hr. **Bronchospasm:** 2 mg nebulizer q 6 hrs.

---

[166] Bevan DR, et al, "Reversal of neuromuscular blockade," Anesthesiology, 1992;77(4):785-805.

Adverse effects: Paradoxical bradycardia for dose < 0.5 mg. Tachycardia may cause myocardial ischemia. Delirium. Mydriasis. Urinary retention. May exacerbate intestinal ileus or obstruction, myasthenia gravis.

Beta-Adrenergic Blockers [167]

See individual entries for esmol I, labetalol, metoprolol, propranolol.

Action and indications: Antagonize circulating catecholamines. β-1-adrenergic activity: cardiac inotropy, chronotropy, dromotropy, lusitropy, vasoconstriction; β-2 effect: visceral smooth muscle relaxation including pulmonary bronchioles. Used to suppress angina, dysrhythmias, hypertension, anxiety, tremor, thyrotoxicosis, aortic dissection, pheochromocytoma crisis, reduce MI size, and postinfarction cardiac death. **Endpoint:** usually pulse 55-60 on mild exertion.

Adverse effects: Bronchospasm, bradycardia, AV block, hypotension, CHF, hypoglycemia in diabetics especially ESRD, depression, fatigue. May exacerbate peripheral vascular insufficiency.

Relative contraindications: CHF (although investigational role in cardiomyopathy), hypotension/shock, AV block or PR>240ms, COPD/asthma, severe diabetes (masks tachycardia), Raynaud, peripheral vascular disease, allergic rhinitis.

Caution: Myasthenia gravis. MAO inhibitors in past 2 weeks. Use care in ischemic LV dysfunction; Treat β-blocker-induced CHF with dig, beta-agonists, glucagon, atropine. Sudden discontinuation can exacerbate angina or ischemia. Do not use as monotherapy in suspected α- and β-adrenergic crises, eg pheochromocytoma or severe cocaine toxicity; combine with α-blocker or use labetalol. Additive AV block with diltiazem, verapamil, digoxin.

Comparative properties:

Name	β-1[a]	ISA	MSA[c]	Lipid[d]	T½ hr normal/ESRD[e]	Adjust for GFR: >50 / 10-50 / <10	Typical Dosage range (mg)
Acebutolol	+	+	Ia	0.52	7-9 / 7	100 / 50 / 30-50%	200-600 bid
Atenolol	+	-		0.06	7 / 15-35	100/ 50 / 30-50%	25-200 qd
Betaxolol	+	-		Low	14-22 / ?	—	10-40 qd
Carteolol	-	+		Low	7 / 33	100/ 50 / 25%	2.5-10 qd
Esmolol	+	-		—	0.13 / 0.13	—	
Labetalol[f]	-	-	Ia		3-9 / 3-9	—	100-1200 bid
Metoprolol	+	-		0.59	3.5/2.5-4.5	—	25-200 bid
Nadolol	-	-		0.19	19 / 45	100/ 50 / 25%	40-240 qd
Pindolol	-	+	Ia	0.48	3-4 / 3-4	—	5-30 bid
Propranolol	-	-	Ia	1.0	2-6 / 1-6	—	10-160 qid
Sotalol	-	-	III	?	7.5-15/56	100 / 30 / 15-30%	80-320 bid
Timolol	-	-		0.57	2.7 / 4	—	10-20 bid

a: β-1 specificity b: ISA = Intrinsic sympathomimetic activity (partial β-1 agonism), may ↓bradycardia & negative inotropy, but no survival benefit in post-MI pts, unlike agents without ISA. c: MSA = Membrane stabilizing activity = class IA antiarrhythmic properties, of uncertain significance. Sotalol has class III antiarrhythmic properties. d: Lipid solubility, as a fraction of propranolol. e: Biological exceeds pharmacological half-life. f: Labetalol has both α- and β-adrenergic antagonist properties.

Bicarbonate

Action: Systemic or urinary alkalinizing agent. Used in hyperkalemia (transiently shifts potassium intracellularly), severe metabolic acidosis, intoxications with tricyclic antidepressants, phenobarbital, cocaine, in diuresis of drugs like salicylates and of nephrotoxic agents like uric acid & myoglobin. Limited benefits (see below). Note ventilation is the primary therapy of respiratory acidosis;

[167] BB Hoffman & RJ Lefkowitz, "Adrenergic receptor antagonists," in Goodman & Gilman's Pharmacologic basis of therapeutics, 8/e, p 234, 1990.

restoring adequate perfusion the primary therapy of metabolic (lactic) acidosis from tissue hypoperfusion.

Caution: Multiple adverse effects: induces paradoxical intracellular acidosis by liberating CO_2 which crosses cell membrane more freely than HCO_3; shifts oxyhemoglobin saturation curve and reduces O_2 delivery; induces hypernatremia and hyperosmolality; may precipitate exogenously-administered catecholamines.

Kinetics: Distributed in total body water = $0.6 \times$ weight.

IV: **Hyperkalemia, urgent intractable acidosis:** Sodium bicarbonate 1 mEq/kg bolus (1 amp = 50 mEq) then 0.5-1.0 mEq/kg q 10 minutes as guided by arterial blood gas analysis. **Note** bicarbonate is distributed in total body water = $0.6 \times$ body weight. Typical desired bicarbonate $\geq$ 18 mEq/L. **Bicarbonate deficit** (mEq) = (Desired · Actual HCO_3 mEq/L) × 0.6 L/kg × body weight kg. **Urinary alkalinization:** 2-5 mEq/kg IV over 4-8hr, mix 3 amps $NaHCO_3$ in 1 liter D5W = 150 mEq/L.

Adverse effects: (See "Caution") Volume overload, hypercapnea, alkalemia, hyperosmolarity, hypocalcemia, hypokalemia.

Bretylium tosylate[168]

Action: Second-line class III antiarrhythmic for VT/VF unresponsive to defib/epi/lidocaine/procainamide. Elevates VF threshold. Accumulates in sympathetic ganglionic & postganglionic adrenergic neurons to block norepinephrine (NE) release & reuptake. Biphasic action: initial ~20-minutes induces neuronal NE release, causing transient NE tachycardia, hypertension. Subsequently inhibits peripheral neuronal NE release, peaking at 45-60 min, causing hypotension, especially postural.

Kinetics: Pure renal elimination unchanged. Onset 15-20 min, peak 45-60 min, note "paradoxical" sympathomimetic initial 20 min. $T\frac{1}{2}$ 6-14 hrs, ESRD 16-32 hrs.

Dose: **V-Fib:** 5mg/kg undiluted $\Rightarrow$ shock $\Rightarrow$ 10mg/kg q 15-30 min to max 30 mg/kg. **V-Tach:** mix 500 mg in 50 mL D5W, 5-10 mg/kg over 8-10 min and repeat once. Infuse 1-2mg/min or intermittent 5-10mg/kg over 10-30 min q 6-8 hr.

Renal failure: GFR 10-50: 25-50%, GFR < 10: 25% dose. Not dialyzed.

Caution: Hypotension, nausea, vomiting especially with rapid infusion in awake patient. Initially, keep supine, may require IV fluids or pressors. Chronic use may induce postdenervation hypersensitivity, may become very catecholamine-sensitive. Digitalis toxicity may be exacerbated by initial catecholamine surge. Accumulates in renal failure. Monitor for QT, > 0.5s.

Interactions: May $\uparrow$ catecholamine sensitivity and aggravate dig toxicity.

Calcium

Indications: Hypocalcemia (eg posttransfusion), reverse calcium channel blocker mediated hypotension, "protect" against hyperkalemic arrhythmias. No likely benefit in pulseless electrical activity.

PO: Calcium carbonate 40% Ca; gluconate 9% Ca.

IV: 2-4 mg/kg Ca as necessary q 10 min.
Calcium chloride 1Amp/1g/10mL of 10% = 272mg/13.6mEq Ca.
Calcium gluconate 1Amp/1g/10mL of 10% = 90mg/4.5mEq Ca is less irritating.
Calcium 20 mg = 1 mMol = 1 mEq. Infusion: 10mL of 10% CaCl in 500mL over 6hrs. **Acute hyperkalemia:** 10-20mL of 10% CaCl, IV over 1-5 min, may repeat. **Tetany** usually requires 200mg Ca to abort, given IV over 10 min.

Caution: Arrhythmogenic with digoxin. Severe desiccant. Causes bradycardia, paresthesias, hypercalcemia. Don't mix with phosphate, sulfate, carbonates. Correct hypokalemia before hypocalcemia. Note concomitant hypomagnesemia common in hypocalcemia.

---

[168] ACLS; J Anderson, "Bretylium tosylate," in Messerli FH(ed.) Cardiovascular Drug Therapy, Philadelphia: Saunders, 1990.

Chlorothiazide *(Diuril)*

<u>Action</u>: Parenteral thiazide diuretic useful in overcoming diuretic "resistance" in refractory volume overload, combined with loop diuretics.

<u>Kinetics</u>: Onset 15 min, peak 30 min, T½ 45-120 min, renal excretion.

<u>IV</u>: 500-1000 mg IV along with furosemide or bumetanide, q 12-24hr.

Clonidine *(Catapres)*

<u>Action</u>: Central α-2 adrenergic agonist reduces peripheral sympathetic activity, causes vasodilation and vagally-mediated bradycardia, decreased renin-angiotensin-aldosterone activity, no reduction of renal blood flow. Used as hypotensive, to diagnose pheochromocytoma (does not suppress plasma NE unlike benign hyperadrenergic states), management of opiate/EtOH withdrawal, migraine prophylaxis, may ↓ portal HTN.

<u>Kinetics</u>: T½ 6-20 hrs, 18-41 ESRD. Liver metabolism. Onset 30-60 min after po dose, max effect 2-3 hrs.

<u>PO</u>: **Urgent HTN**: 0.1-0.2 mg then 0.1 mg hourly until 0.5 mg or target BP. **Chronic HTN**: 0.1 mg bid, ↑ 0.1mg/dose/wk; usual range 0.2-0.6 bid.

<u>Renal failure</u>: No adjustment.

<u>Cutaneous patch</u>: Apply weekly, total daily po dose, steady-state after 2-3d.

<u>Caution</u>: **Withdrawal** syndrome uncommon 24-72 hrs after stopping, usually sympathetic hyperactivity with ↑ BP overshoot. Care especially in angina or with β-blockers. Withdraw β-blockers first.

<u>Side effects</u>: Dry mouth (~50%), drowsy (~30%), sedation (~8%), postural hypotension (3%) constipation, urinary retention, impotence, usually abate 4-6 wks, uncommon in patch. Contact dermatitis from patch.

<u>Interactions</u>: ↓'d efficacy with TCA's, MOAI's. Exacerbates sedative effects of other drugs.

Corticosteroids

Potency (mg equivalents to cortisol)	Glucocorticoid	Mineralocorticoid
Short-acting (biological half-life <12h)		
Cortisol (Hydrocortisone)	1	1
Cortisone acetate[169]	0.8	0.8
Intermediate (biological half-life 12-36h)		
Aldosterone	0.1	400
Fludrocortisone *(Florinef)*	10	400
Prednisone	4	0.25
Prednisolone	4	0.25
Methylprednisolone	5	<0.01
Triamcinolone	5	<0.01
Long (biological half-life > 48h)		
Betamethasone	25	<0.01
Dexamethasone	30-40	<0.01

<u>Dosage</u>: **"Stress-dose"**: hydrocortisone 100 mg IV q 6-8hrs. **Addisonian crisis**: same as "stress dose" + volume repletion. **Adrenal replacement therapy**: hydrocortisone 12-15 mg/m²/day, two-thirds in AM, one-third in PM. **Bronchospasm**: Methylprednisolone 60-120 mg IV then 40-60 mg q 6 hrs. **Cerebral edema**: dexamethasone 10 mg IV then 4-6 mg q 4-6 hrs. **Acute spinal injury**: Methylprednisolone 30 mg/kg IV then infuse 5.4 mg/kg/hr x 23 hrs.

---

[169] Requires hepatic metabolism of prodrug into cortisol; poorly absorbed and metabolized given IM/SQ.

Dantrolene[170]

Action: Direct skeletal (not cardiac or smooth) muscle relaxation, interferes with calcium release from sarcoplasmic reticulum. Used to treat malignant hyperthermia, along with oxygen, cooling, and correction of acidosis. Possible role in neuroleptic malignant syndrome.

Kinetics: Onset rapid. Half-life 4-8 hrs after IV.

Dose: 1-2 mg/kg rapid IV. Repeat rapidly as necessary until reversal of process (usually 2.5mg/kg) or maximum 10mg/kg. Follow with 4-8mg/kg daily in 4 divided doses po for 3 days.

Interactions: Verapamil combined causes marked cardiac depression. Potentiates nondepolarizing neuromuscular blockers.

Desmopressin (ddAVP)[171]

Action: Synthetic vasopressin analog, used to replace ADH, to control hemorrhage in uremia, hemophilia A (when factor VIII activity > 5%), and von Willebrand disease. Induces endothelial release of von Willebrand Factor and hepatic factor VIII release.

Kinetics: Bleeding time minimized in 1-2 hrs, effect persists ~4hrs.

Dosage: **Hemorrhage:** 0.3 μg/kg SQ or IV (mixed in 50mL NS) over 20-30 min. Administer 30 min before surgery. Consider **adjunctive** transfusion to Hct>25%, conjugated estrogen 0.6 mg/kg IV (onset hrs-days). If life-threatening, consider cryoprecipitate 10 bags IV[172]. **Central diabetes insipidus:** 10-40 μg qd-bid nasal spray titrated to urine output & plasma sodium. Nasal 10× less potent than IV/SQ.

Caution: Tachyphylaxis may occur after 24-48 hrs continuous usage, possibly related to vWF depletion.

Side effects: Water intoxication, platelet-aggregation & thrombosis, myocardial ischemia, hypotension with rapid infusion, abdominal distress.

Digoxin

Action & Kinetics: Bradycardia by enhancing vagal tone; Weak inotrope by inhibiting Na-K-ATPase and ↑ing cytosolic Ca. Reduces CHF hospital admissions without mortality effect. $T_{1/2}$ 36-44 hrs, ESRD 80-120 hrs. Renal clearance, 18-28% cleared by stool, liver. Loading dose saturates skeletal muscle receptors. Onset 20-30 min IV; 2hrs po.

Dosing: "**Digitalization:**" Ideal 0.9 mg/m² BSA per 24hrs; Practically 1-2mg in divided doses over 2 days: typically 0.5mg IV then 0.25mg IV/po q 6hrs. **Rate control** in afib[173]: HR>160: 0.375-0.5 mg IV; HR 140-160: 0.25-0.375 mg IV; HR 120-140: 0.25 mg IV; HR 110-120: 0.125 mg IV. Redose prn q 1-4hrs. **Maintenance:** 0.1-0.5mg/d, typically 0.25mg qd. Adjust for GFR: typically 0.125 mg/d for CL_{CR} < 50.

Renal failure: Halve load. GFR>50: 100% q 24h; GFR 10-50: 25-75% q 36h; GFR<10: 10-25% dose q 48h. CAVH supplement 0.5 mg q 12h. See "levels."

Contraindications: Hypertrophic cardiomyopathy; significant AV block; Wolff-Parkinson-White with possible antegrade conduction. Relative contraindications: cardioversion, risk of toxicity incl cor pulmonale; diastolic LV dysfunction.

Levels: Therapeutic 1-2ng/mL for CHF, higher (2-4ng/mL) for SVTs. Toxicity may occur at low levels, esp. acutely. Levels unhelpful in afib (endpoints: VR & toxicity). Measure column-separated digoxin levels in ESRD.

---

[170] Wedel DJ, et al, "Clinical effects of intravenously administered dantrolene," Mayo Clin Proc, 1995;70(3):241-6; Guze BH; Baxter LR Jr, "Current concepts. Neuroleptic malignant syndrome," N Engl J Med, 1985;313(3):163-6.

[171] PM Manucci, et al, "Deamino-8-d-arginine vasopressin shortens the bleeding time in uremia," N Engl J Med 1983;308:8-12.

[172] ME Eberst & LR Berkowitz, "Hemostasis in renal disease," Am J Med, 1994;96(2):168.

[173] A Waldo & WAH MacLean, Diagnosis and treatment of cardiac arrhythmias following open heart surgery, Futura, 1983; p 214.

Toxicity: Anorexia, nausea, vomiting, diarrhea, malaise, fatigue, confusion, facial pain, insomnia, depression, vertigo, green/yellow halo around lights; palpitation, syncope; hyperkalemia.

Interactions: **High digoxin level:** Quinidine, verapamil, diltiazem, amiodarone, propafenone, trimethoprim (↑ed clearance), K-retaining diuretics (spironolactone, amiloride, triamterene), ↓ed enteric bacterial breakdown (erythromycin, tetracycline), ↓ed renal blood flow (beta-blockers, CHF), severe hypokalemia, sulfonylureas, anticholinergics (↑ed absorption), hydroxychloroquine, hypothyroidism, ? cimetidine, ? flecainide. **Low digoxin level:** ↓ed absorption (GI edema, hyperthyroidism, antacids, cholestyramine, metoclopramide, sulfasalazine, neomycin); Clearance↑: (ACE inhibitors, nitroprusside, hydralazine, phenytoin, rifampin).

Digoxin Immune Fab[174] *(Digibind)*

Indication: **Life-threatening** digoxin toxicity, typically arrhythmia, digoxin level>10. Hyperkalemia portends imminent cardiac arrest, is an indication.

Action: Affinity of digoxin for Digibind is greater than for Na,K-ATPase. Fab has large volume of distribution.

IV: Dose (in # of vials) = (Serum digoxin level ng/mL)×(weight in kg)/100. Give IV over 30 minutes or bolus if necessary.

Caution: K levels may drop precipitously after administration. May precipitate acute CHF. Digoxin toxicity may also require potassium, lidocaine, phenytoin, procainamide, propranolol, atropine, pacemaker. Renal failure may cause spuriously elevated digoxin levels by certain assays.

Contraindications: Hx sensitivity to sheep products, previous Fab.

Diltiazem IV[175] *(Cardizem)*

Action: Slow Ca-channel-antagonist, prolongs AV nodal refractoriness. Used IV to slow ventricular response to atrial fibrillation or flutter, to interrupt SVTs involving AV node, and to control rest angina. Lowers BP by relaxing vascular smooth muscle without significant reflex tachycardia. Negative inotrope.

Kinetics[176]: IV response time 5 min, peak 11 min. Plasma elimination half-life 3.4 hrs. Cytochrome P450 degradation.

IV: **Tachycardias** 0.25 mg/kg given over 2 min (average 20 mg). If unsatisfactory response, after 15 min give 0.35 mg/kg over 2 min. Continuous infusion **mix** 250 mL solution + 250 mL fluid = 0.833 mg/mL, infuse 5-15 mg/hr. **Transition to po** agent after 3 hrs.

Renal failure: No adjustment.

Contraindications: Undiagnosed wide-complex tachycardia!, WPW, 2° AV block or higher, sick-sinus syndrome, low BP, concurrent β-blockers.

Side-effects: Hypotension, high-degree AV block, biochemical hepatitis, flushing, injection site reaction.

Pregnancy: Class C.

Dobutamine[177]

Action: Racemic mixture: L-isomer is alpha-1 agonist, D-isomer is nonspecific beta-agonist. Reduces SVR as it increases inotropy. No dopaminergic activity. Hemodynamic effect comparable to dopamine + nitroprusside. Less chronotropy than isoproterenol. Onset 1-2 min, peak effect 5-10min, half-life 2.4 minutes.

Renal failure: No dose adjustment.

---

[174] Hickey AR; *et al*, "Digoxin Immune Fab therapy in the management of digitalis intoxication: safety and efficacy results of an observational surveillance study," *J Am Coll Cardiol*, 1991;17(3):590-8.

[175] Goldenberg IF, *et al*, "Intravenous diltiazem for the treatment of patients with atrial fibrillation or flutter and moderate to severe congestive heart failure," *Am J Cardiol*, 1994;74(9):884-9.

[176] Dias VC, *et al*, "Pharmacokinetics and pharmacodynamics of intravenous diltiazem in patients with atrial fibrillation or atrial flutter," *Circulation*, 1992;86(5):1421-8.

[177] Chatterjee K, *et al*, "Dobutamine in heart failure," *Eur Heart J*, 1982;3(Suppl D):107-14; Leier CV, Unverferth DV, "Drugs five years later. Dobutamine," *Ann Intern Med*, 1983;99(4):490-6.

Uses: Inotrope, for acute circulatory failure from decreased myocardial contractility, eg MI, severe acute CHF decompensation, cardiac surgery. Also increases CO in RV infarct unresponsive to volume.

IV: Mix 250mg in 500mL D5W = 500μg/mL beginning at 0.5μg/ kg/min (4.2mL/hr for 70kg man). Usual range 2.5-20μg/kg/min. Maximum 40μg/kg/min.

Caution: Enhances AV conduction especially in atrial fibrillation. May precipitate or exacerbate ventricular arrhythmia.

Contraindications: Hypertrophic cardiomyopathy.

Incompatibility: Alkali (theophylline, bicarbonate).

Dopamine

Action: At low doses (1-2μg/kg/min) produces renal, mesenteric, cerebral vasodilation via dopaminergic receptors without cardiac effects. At intermediate range (2-10μg/kg/min) stimulates beta-1 and alpha-adrenergic receptors, acting as inotrope and vasopressor. At high doses (>10μg/kg/min) acts predominantly as alpha-agonist vasoconstrictor. These dose ranges must be individualized.

Indications: As an inotrope, especially in combination with nitroprusside (net hemodynamic effect resembling dobutamine). As a vasopressor for hypotension in the absence of hypovolemia. To improve renal blood flow, especially at low doses along with a vasopressor, as in septic shock.

IV: Mix 400 mg in 250 mL D5W = 1.6mg/mL beginning at 1μg/kg/min (2.6mL/hr for 70 kg pt). If using "renal dose" DA, titrate to vital signs before infusion and at each dose; ↑ HR and ↑ BP imply "renal dose" is exceeded. Vasopressor effect generally limited at doses > 40μg/kg/min; consider switching to norepinephrine.

Caution: Start with 10% of dose in pts with circulating MAO inhibitors. Avoid cyclopropane or halogenated hydrocarbon anesthetics. Enhances AV conduction especially in atrial fibrillation. DA agonists may exacerbate psychoses. Treat extravasation aggressively as with norepinephrine (see phentolamine page 117).

Incompatibility: Alkali (bicarbonate, theophylline) inactivate dopamine. Nevertheless this interaction is slow enough that drugs may coinfuse in a single catheter.

Pregnancy: Class C.

Edrophonium *(Tensilon)*

Action: Rapid-acting anticholinesterase used to diagnose myasthenia gravis (MG) or to increase vagal tone; effect 30-60 sec; duration 10 min.

Positive Test: Increase in muscle strength (ptosis, diplopia, respiration, dysphonia/phagia/arthria, limb strength) but absent adverse reactions like fasciculations (orbicularis oculi, facial muscles, limb muscles) and side effects (lacrimation, diaphoresis, salivation, cramps, N/V/D).

Adverse Reactions: Eye: lacrimation, diplopia, spasm of accommodation, pupillary constriction. CNS: seizure, dysarthria, dysphonia, dysphagia. Resp: Secretions, bronchoconstriction, hypoventilation. Cardiac: bradycardia, vagal hypotension. GI: Salivation, gastric & intestinal secretions and peristalsis, N/V/D. Skeletal weakness & fasciculations. Urinary incontinence.

Dosage: 10mg (1mL) in tuberculin syringe. Keep **atropine** available. Give 2mg (0.2mL) IV. Only if no adverse reaction in 45 seconds, give remainder of doses; otherwise give atropine 0.5mg IV. To test for adequacy of MG drugs, give 1-2mg one hour after po drugs.

Warning: Treat overdose with respiratory care, atropine, pralidoxime, cardiac monitoring, antiseizure measures.

Enalaprilat *(Vasotec IV)*

Action: Angiotensin converting enzyme inhibitor, active metabolite of orally-administered prodrug enalapril. Used as parenteral hypotensive. Not generally used as afterload reducer in absence of hypertension.

IV: 0.625-1.25 mg over 5 min q 6 hr, response in 15 min, may repeat 0.625 mg in 1 hr if response inadequate. Use lower dose in patients on diuretics. Max 5 mg q 6

hr. Manufacturer suggests this protocol regardless of oral enalapril dose; 1.25 mg IV ≈ 5 mg po enalapril.
Renal failure: Dose 0.625 mg IV q 6 hr for CL_{cr}< 30 mL/min.
Side-effects: Hypotension especially in intravascular volume depletion; reduced GFR in renal insufficiency & renovascular disease; hyperkalemia; angioedema; agranulocytosis; cough; reversible renal failure in bilateral renal artery stenosis.
Pregnancy: Contraindicated, fetal morbidity & mortality in 3rd trimester.

Epinephrine[178] (Adrenalin)

Action: Nonspecific adrenergic agonist; has β-2 activity unlike norepinephrine (NE). Compared to NE twice as potent inotrope & chronotrope, equipotent vasopressor. At low doses (< 4 μg/kg/min), α effects less important; β-2 mediated vasodilator with compensatory increase in cardiac output. Potent bronchodilator.
Indications: Cardiac arrest, anaphylaxis, severe bronchospasm & laryngospasm, cardiogenic shock especially post cardiac surgery.
IV: **Cardiac arrest:** 1 mg (10mL of 1:10,000) q 3-5 min IV bolus followed by 20 mL flush, or infusion mix 30 mg in 250 mL fluid begin @ 100 mL/h, or endotracheal 2.5 mg q 3-5 min. Limited data support bolus doses of 3-5 mg IV q 3-5 min. **High dose for asystole:** 0.1 mg/kg IV q3-5 min. **Shock:** Mix 4 mg in 250ml D5W=16 μg/mL. Start 2μg/min, titrate to effect up to ~20 μg/min. **Note** α-effects predominate >4μg/min.
Subcutaneous: **Bronchospasm & anaphylaxis:** 0.1 mg SQ, equivalent to 20 μg/min IV. Local vasoconstriction reduces absorption.
Adverse effects: Increased myocardial oxygen demand, tachyarrhythmias, decreased splanchnic perfusion, HTN, ↑Glc, ↓K, CNS activation.
Interactions: MAOIs, TCAs dramatically potentiate activity. Halothane anesthetics "sensitize" myocardium to arrhythmias. **Incompatible** with bicarbonate but may coinfuse.

Epoprostenol[179] (Flolan) (Prostacyclin, Prostaglandin I₂)

Action: Short-acting vasodilator with diverse effects, inhibits platelet aggregation. Prolongs survival in primary pulmonary hypertension, generally used as a bridge to transplantation.
Kinetics: Rapid hydrolysis in blood, T½ 6 minutes.
IV: Initial dose guided by PA catheter and pulse-oximetry: 2 ng/kg/min, increment by 2 ng/kg/min q 15 min until intolerable side effects, MAP declines 40%, HR increases 40%. Continuous infusion pump available[180]. Dosage requirements increase over time to 20-200ng/kg/min.
Side-effects: Hypotension, nausea, vomiting, headache, flushing, lightheadedness, restlessness, anxiety, abdominal pain, dyspnea, tachycardia, bradycardia.
Caution: Exacerbates R → L shunting across patent foramen ovale can worsen hypoxemia.

Esmolol (Brevibloc)

Action & kinetics: β1-selective, T½ 9 min, distribution time 2 min. Steady-state 5 min with load, 30 min without. β-blockade remits 10-20 min after stopping. Esterified in RBCs. Slows AV node conduction. Used in atrial flutter, a-fib, inappropriate sinus-tach[181]. Combine with nitroprusside for aortic dissection; combine with phentolamine for pheochromocytoma crisis or thyroid storm. Reduces myocardial

---

[178] Goodman & Gilman's Pharmacologic basis of therapeutics, 8th edition, 1990; ACLS guidelines.
[179] RJ Barst, et al, "A comparison of continuous intravenous epoprostenol (prostacyclin) with conventional therapy for primary pulmonary hypertension," N Engl J Med 1996; 334(5):296-301. "Epoprostenol," Med Lett Drugs Ther 1996; 38(968):14-15.
[180] Quantum Health Resources is sole distributor 1-800-9-FLOLAN.
[181] Byrd RC, et al, "Safety and efficacy of esmolol (an ultrashort-acting beta-adrenergic blocking agent) for control of ventricular rate in supraventricular tachycardias," J Am Coll Cardiol, 1984;3(2 Pt 1):394-9.

ischemia[182] but more hypotensive than other β-blockers[183]. Particularly useful to test tolerability of β-blockers in patients with relative contraindications.

IV: **Mix** 5g in 500mL D5W = 10mg/mL. **Load** 500µg/kg over one minute then 50µ g/kg/min. Titrate q 4 minutes reloading each time, increase infusion by 50µ g/kg/min each time. As target HR approaches, skip load with titration. Maximum 200 µg/kg/min (one use up to 300µg/kg/min).

Renal failure: Half-life unchanged. No dose adjustment.

Transition to alternative agent: 30 minutes after 1st dose of dig/verap/propranolol, ↓ infusion 50%. If satisfactory 60min after 2nd dose of (agent), DC infusion.

Caution: Bronchospasm, DM. IV irritant, don't use butterfly, avoid extravasation, use concentration < 10mg/mL. NaHCO₃ incompatible.

Adverse interactions: Additive effect with reserpine.

Side effects: Pallor, nausea, flushing, brady, CP, pulm edema, asystole.

Ethanol[184]

Action: Competitive substrate for alcohol dehydrogenase to limit toxic metabolites of ingested methanol & ethylene glycol. Target levels 100-150 mg/dl, must be checked frequently along with glucose. **Conversions:** specific gravity EtOH is 0.79 mg/mL. 10% IV = EtOH 7.9 g/dL. 86 proof whisky = EtOH 34 g/dL.

Load: 800 mg/kg (based on EtOH level 0) giving blood EtOH ≅ 100 mg/dL.

IV: Loading dose as 5-10% in water, or 500 mL 10% ethanol in H₂O over 1hr.

PO: Four 30mL (1 oz) shots of 80 proof liquor for 70 kg patient, or loading dose as 20-30% ethanol in water.

Maintenance: 130 mg/kg/hr and titrate to levels ≅ 100 mg/dL. Give 250-350 mg/kg/hr if patient is a chronic alcoholic, while on hemodialysis, or if charcoal is given. EtOH causes hypoglycemia during prolonged infusion.

Caution: Also administer folic acid 50 mg IV q 4 hr.

Flumazenil[185] *(Romazicon)*

Action: Competitive antagonist of benzodiazepines at the GABA_A/benzo receptor. Used to diagnose benzodiazepine intoxication, and to reverse sedation & respiratory depression from benzodiazepines.

IV: **Known isolated benzodiazepine overdose:** 0.2 mg over 30 sec. If still lethargic give 0.3 mg over 30 sec. May repeat 0.5 mg over 30 sec q minute to maximum 3 mg. May rebolus 0.5 mg/hr to maintain wakefulness. Benzo intoxication unlikely if no response after 5 mg. **Reversal of conscious sedation:** 0.2 mg over 15 sec, if sedated after 45 sec give 0.2 mg IV. Repeat q 1 min up to total 1 mg.

Kinetics: Metabolized by liver. Elimination half-time ~50-60 min if liver normal.

Caution: May provoke withdrawal syndrome including seizures in chronic benzo abusers and in suspected tricyclic antidepressant overdose. Half-life of benzos may exceed that of flumazenil. Sedation may be reversed earlier than is respiratory depression.

Side-effects: Agitation, myoclonus, nausea, vomiting.

Fosphenytoin *(Cerebyx IV)*
See Phenytoin on page 118.

---

[182] Kirshenbaum JM; et al, "Use of an ultrashort-acting beta-receptor blocker (esmolol) in patients with acute myocardial ischemia and relative contraindications to beta-blockade therapy," J Am Coll Cardiol. 1988;12(3):773-80.

[183] Deegan R; Wood AJ, "Beta-receptor antagonism does not fully explain esmolol-induced hypotension," Clin Pharm Ther, 1994;56(2):223-8.

[184] LR Goldfrank et al, "Methanol, ethylene glycol, and isopropenol," in Goldfrank's Toxicologic emergencies, 4th ed, (1990), pp 481-497.

[185] "Flumazenil," Med Lett Drugs Ther, 1992; 34(874):66-8. Hoffman RS; Goldfrank LR, "The poisoned patient with altered consciousness. Controversies in the use of a 'coma cocktail'," Jama, 1995;274(7):562-9; Shapiro BA, et al, "Practice parameters for intravenous analgesia and sedation for adult patients in the intensive care unit: an executive summary. Society of Critical Care Medicine," Crit Care Med, 1995;23(9):1596-600.

Glucagon [186]

Action: Peptide hormone stimulates hepatic glycogenolysis and gluconeogenesis, ↓ glycogen synthesis, ↑ lipolysis; part of insulin counterregulatory system. Used as hyperglycemic. Used as GI smooth muscle relaxant transiently to decrease motility. In suprahysiologic doses it is a positive inotrope, probably by activating cAMP independently of adrenergic receptors; used in hypotension/bradycardia unresponsive to catecholamines, especially after overdose of calcium-channel· or β-adrenergic· antagonists. Inotrope > chronotrope.

Kinetics: Half-life 3-6 minutes, onset 1 min, comparable to insulin.

IV: **Hypoglycemia:** 0.5-1mg IV/IM/SQ, may repeat q 15 min 1-2 times, use glucose if necessary. **Hypotension/bradycardia:** 5-10 mg bolus then 1-5mg/hr infusion.

Caution: Hepatic glucose stores are rapidly depleted in **fasting**/starved patients or those with **liver disease**; use glucose instead. Promotes insulin release in **insulinoma** with resultant hypoglycemia. Elicits catecholamine release by **pheochromocytoma** (treat with **phentolamine**).

Haloperidol [187] (Haldol)

Action: Antipsychotic and sedative via dopaminergic blockade. Does not depress respiratory drive.

Kinetics: Half-life 12-38 hrs. Liver metabolism.

IV/IM: **Acute psychosis & severe agitation:** 2-5 mg q 20-30 min until symptoms abate, usually < 10-15 mg total [188]. May give IV over 2-3 min [188]. Active psychosis: 0.5-5 mg po/IM bid-tid. **Agitation in elderly or debilitated:** 0.5-2 mg po qd, increment 0.5mg.

Renal failure: Half-life unknown. No dosage adjustment. Not dialyzed.

Caution: Reduce dose in liver (extreme case) and renal failure. Thyrotoxicosis profoundly exacerbates extrapyramidal effects. High doses may cause *Torsades de Pointes* (polymorphic VT).

Side-effects: Anticholinergic, extrapyramidal, orthostatic hypotension. Neuroleptic malignant syndrome, tardive dyskinesia (risk greater in elderly with prolonged higher-dose therapy), leukopenia, rash, hyperprolactinemia.

Pregnancy: Suspected teratogen in 1st trimester.

Heparin [189] (Unfractionated)

Action: Accelerates antithrombin III inhibition of factors II (thrombin), IX, X, XI & XII, thereby inhibiting thrombin-induced activation of factors V and VIII. Anticoagulant in treatment/prophylaxis of thrombosis & thromboembolism, coronary syndromes, and catheter flushes.

Kinetics: Anticoagulation increases disproportionately with increasing dose. Biological T½ 30 min after 25U/kg bolus, but T½ 60 min after 75U/kg. No important difference among bovine, porcine, sodium or calcium heparins.

IV: **Venous thromboembolism:** 80 U/kg IV then 18 U/kg-hr **or** 5000U IV then 1250 U/hr or 17,500U SQ q 12hrs. Adjust 6 hrs afterwards for APTT 1.5-2.5 × control. **Prevention of venous thromboembolism:** 5000U SQ q 12hrs. High-risk pts should have dose adjusted to increase APTT to upper-normal limits. **Unstable**

[186] K Hall-Boyer, et al, "Glucagon: hormone or therapeutic agent?" Crit Care Med, 1984;12:584.

[187] Riker RR; et al, "Continuous infusion of haloperidol controls agitation in critically ill patients," Crit Care Med, 1994;22(3):433-40; Shapiro BA, et al, "Practice parameters for intravenous analgesia and sedation for adult patients in the intensive care unit: an executive summary. Society of Critical Care Medicine," Crit Care Med, 1995;23(9):1596-600.

[188] The US FDA does not approve haloperidol for IV administration. The decanoate preparation is unsuitable for IV administration.

[189] Hirsh J, et al, "Heparin: mechanism of action, pharmacokinetics, dosing considerations, monitoring, efficacy, and safety," Chest 1995;108(4 Suppl):258S-275S. Raschke RA, et al, "The weight-based heparin dosing nomogram compared with a standard care nomogram. A randomized controlled trial," Ann Intern Med 1993;119(9):874-81.

angina: 80 U/kg IV then 18 U/kg-hr **Myocardial infarction with tPA:** 5000U IV then 1000 U/hr. Weight-based full dosing ↑es hemorrhagic stroke after tPA[190]. Add aspirin in MI.

<u>Renal failure</u>: Half-life unchanged. No dosage adjustment.

<u>Dosage adjustment</u>:

APTT (sec)	Rebolus	Stop	Δ infusion	Next APTT
< 35s (<1.2×control)	80 u/kg	-	↑ 4u/kg-hr	6 hr
35-45s (1.2-1.5×control)	40 u/kg	-	↑ 2u/kg-hr	6 hr
46-70s (1.5-2.3×control)	-	-	-	Next AM
71-90s (2.3-3×control)	-	-	↓ 2u/kg-hr	Next AM
> 90s (>3×control)	0	60 min	↓ 3u/kg-hr	6 hr

<u>Adverse effects</u>: Hemorrhage, esp. in seriously ill, alcohol abusers, ? intermittent dosing, aspirin in periop pts. Thrombocytopenia (? porcine lung > porcine gut heparin) after 3-15 days. Thrombosis via platelet aggregation. Osteoporosis after chronic use. Hypoaldosteronism (Type IV RTA) especially in renal insufficiency & diabetes.

<u>Interactions</u>: Nitroglycerin may ↓ heparin effect,[191] (poor study).

<u>Pregnancy</u>: Does not cross placenta; anticoagulant of choice.

Hydralazine *(Apresoline)*

<u>Action</u>: Predominantly arteriolar vasodilator. Reflex tachycardia in healthy subjects, blunted tachycardia in pts with CHF.

<u>Indication</u>: CHF in combination with nitrates; hypertension in combination with diuretic or β-blocker; hypertensive emergencies, esp in pregnancy.

<u>Kinetics</u>: Biological exceeds biochemical $T\frac{1}{2}$ 2-8 hrs. Liver metab (fast-acetylators need 25% more; slow-acetylators more susceptible to lupus-like syndrome).

<u>IV</u>: 5mg (**pregnancy**) or 20mg (**HTN**) then 5-20mg q 20-30min to target BP.

<u>PO</u>: **CHF**: Initial 50 mg bid-qid, up to 600mg/d. **HTN**: Begin 10 mg qid x 2-4d then 25 mg qid then double twice-weekly up to 50-100 mg qid.

<u>Renal failure</u>: $T\frac{1}{2}$ 7-16 hrs. Give q 8-16h for GFR<10. Not dialyzed.

<u>Caution</u>: Slow-acetylators should probably not receive > 200 mg/d.

<u>Side-effects</u>: Lupus syndrome rare < 200mg/day. Renin-release →fluid retention. Reflex tachycardia contraindication in angina. Self-limited HA & nausea on starting tx. B6-sensitive polyneuropathy & drug fever rare.

<u>Pregnancy</u>: Animal not human teratogen. Emergency agent of choice.

Ibutilide[192] *(Corvert)*

<u>Action</u>: Short-acting class III antiarrhythmic used to convert atrial fibrillation or atrial flutter to sinus rhythm. Dose-related QT prolongation is associated with antiarrhythmic activity. Efficacy superior at 90 min to IV procainamide or IV sotalol (both of which may be more efficacious after a longer time interval).

<u>Kinetics</u>: Rapid redistribution terminates drug effect. Elimination $T\frac{1}{2}$ ~6 hr (range 2-12), V_s ~11L/kg, CL ~29mL/min/kg all with high interpatient variability.

<u>IV</u>: **Afib lasting > 48hr**: anticoagulate > 2 wks before cardioversion and 2-4 wks afterwards. **"New" afib or aflutter**: 1.0 mg infused over 10 min (0.01 mg/kg if <60kg). Repeat once if arrhythmia persists 20 min after beginning first infusion. **Continue ECG monitoring ≥ 4 hrs postinfusion.** Consider suppressing pathological rhythm afterwards.

<u>Renal failure</u>: No apparent dosage adjustment warranted. Not studied in liver dz.

<u>Caution</u>: Avoid other antiarrhythmics (especially <u>Class I or Class III</u> agents) before

---

[190] Gusto IIa Investigators, "Randomized trial of intravenous heparin versus recombinant hirudin for acute coronary syndromes," <u>Circulation</u> 1994; 90(4):1631-7.

[191] MA Habbab ,JI Haft, "Heparin resistance induced by intravenous nitroglycerin..." <u>Arch Intern Med</u> 1987;147(5):877.

[192] BS Stambler *et al*, "Efficacy and safety of repeated intravenous doses of ibutilide for rapid conversion of atrial flutter or fibrillation," <u>Circulation</u> 1996;94(7):1613-1621. DM Roden, "Ibutilide and the treatment of atrial arrhythmias," <u>Circulation</u> 1996;94(7):1499-1500.

— and four hours after — administering drug. Avoid in hypokalemia or hypomagnesemia, with QT >440mS or hemodynamically instability. Also untested in decompensated CHF or recent MI. Anticoagulate as appropriate for atrial fibrillation.

Warning: Can cause lethal polymorphic ventricular tachycardia (Torsades de Pointes). 15/180 pts developed polymorphic VT in one study: in 12/15 it resolved spontaneously or with cessation of ibutilide, 3/15 required emergency cardioversion. VT generally begins during or shortly after infusion, and is more common in women, CHF, and those with slower heart rates. Incidence (<2%) of self-limited high-grade AV block and bundle-branch block.

Interactions: Excess risk of Torsades if coadministered with drugs that prolong QT (eg procainamide, quinidine, disopyramide, amiodarone, sotalol, bretylium, tricyclic antidepressants, phenothiazines, H_1-antagonists).

Insulin [193]

Action & kinetics: Anabolic hormone maintains Glc homeostasis: permits Glc translocation, inhibits glycogenolysis & gluconeogenesis, stimulates glycogen synthesis, suppresses lipolysis and ketogenesis, promotes fat synthesis. Drives potassium into cells. Used in hyperglycemia, DKA, acute hyperkalemia. Renal excretion. Plasma half-life 5-9 min.

IV Regular only: Mix 100 units in 100 mL NS or D5W; flush first 10 mL through tubing and waste. Ketoacidosis: 0.1 u/kg/hr, may increase to 0.2-0.3 u/kg/hr if no improvement in acidosis or hyperglycemia in 2-4 hrs. Severe hyperkalemia: Onset in 15-30 min. Give 12-25 units along with dextrose 50% 1-2 amps during first hour. (Give 1 unit insulin for each 2 grams dextrose; D50 1 amp = 50 mL = 25 g.) May rebolus or infuse 40 units insulin in 1 liter 10% dextrose @ 50 mL/hr.

Renal failure: T½ reduced. Give 75% dose if GFR 10-50; 50% if GFR<10.

Subcutaneous insulin preparations:

Insulin	Onset (hrs)	Peak (hrs)	Duration (hrs)
Regular	0.5 -1	2-4	5-7
Semilente	1-2	4-6	12-16
NPH	1-2	6-14	18-26
Lente	1-3	6-14	18-26
Protamine Zinc	6-8	14-24	28-36
Ultralente	6	18-24	28-36

Isoproterenol (Isuprel)

Action & kinetics: Nonspecific β-adrenergic agonist for bradycardia unresponsive to atropine, suppressing Torsades de Pointes. Potent inotrope & chronotrope. Hepatic metabolism. Plasma T½ < 5 min.

IV: Mix 2mg in 250D5W = 8µg/mL. Starting dose 1µg/min (15mL/hr), titrate for effect, up to 10µg/min.

SQ/IM: Undiluted solution 1mL (0.2mg).

Contraindication: Angina/ischemia, digitalis-bradycardia, tachycardias.

Side effects: Hypotension from vasodilatation; tachycardia; ischemia.

Kayexalate (sodium polystyrene sulfonate)

Action: Cation-exchange resin exchanges K^+ for Na^+ in the gut. Treats severe hyperkalemia by removing K from body. Binds ~ 1 mEq K^+ per gram kayexalate. Onset 2-12 hrs po; 30-90 min per rectum.

PO: 15-50 g kayexalate + 30 mL 70% sorbitol q 2-6 hrs.

PR: 50-90 g kayexalate + 50 mL 70% sorbitol + 100 mL water as retention enema q 2-6 hrs followed by cleansing enema; See PDR for details.

Adverse effects: Hypomagnesemia; hypocalcemia; alkalosis; sodium load may

---

[193] American Medical Association, Drug Evaluations, 6th Edition, Chicago: AMA Publications, 1986. Lebovitz HE, "Diabetic ketoacidosis," Lancet, 1995;345(8952):767-72.

precipitate CHF; overshoot hypokalemia; constipation or impaction if used without laxative.

Labetalol[194]

Action: Selective α-1 antagonist, nonselective β-antagonist. α:β 1:3 oral, 1:7 IV. No β-1 agonism (ISA) but may be partial β-2 agonist. Dose-related BP ↓ without reflex brady/tachycardia. Tachyphylaxis uncommon. Used in cocaine intoxication, eclampsia, pheochromocytoma, clonidine withdrawal.

Kinetics: T½ 5-8hrs. Oral onset 2-3 hrs. IV onset 3-5 min. Liver clearance, extensive first-pass metabolism, reduce dose in liver disease.

Renal failure: T½ unchanged. No dosage adjustment. Not dialyzed.

IV: 20mg over 2 minutes then 40-80mg q10min to max 300mg for rapid BP control. Push IV slowly over 2 minutes, **while supine**, then **Infusion** 1-2 mg/min, maximum 2400 mg/day. Stop infusion after satisfactory BP, then repeat q 6-8 hrs. **Mix** 250mg/250ml NS. Change to po by abruptly stopping infusion and waiting for BP to rise.

PO: Initial dose 100 bid, increment 100/dose qd (in-house) or q2-3d (ambulatory). Onset 2-3 hrs. Follow **standing** BP. Usual dose 200-400 bid, max 1200 bid. PO:IV daily total dose 1:1.

Caution: Postural hypotension treated in supine posture. Abrupt discontinuation may precipitate angina, HTN, MI like all beta blockers. Oral beta-predominance may precipitate paradoxical hypertension in pheo and clonidine withdrawal.

Side-effects: Bradycardia, PVD, CHB all less than in pure β-blockers. Postural hypotension, paresthesias, hepatocellular damage, tremor, low-titer insignificant (+) ANA, halothane hypotension.

Pregnancy: Probably safe.

Lidocaine[195]

Action: Class IB antiarrhythmic depresses automaticity, used to suppress ventricular arrhythmia associated with acute ischemia, also as local anesthetic. Not warranted as routine prophylaxis in acute MI.

Kinetics: T½ 1.4hrs initially lengthens to 3hrs with infusions > 1day. T½ increases with: CHF, age, liver disease. Extensive hepatic metabolism to MEGX and GX, which accumulate in renal failure and may cause CNS toxicity. Rapid redistribution of initial load (T½ ~4-8min) requires rebolus.

IV: **Load** 1-1.5 mg/kg over 1-2min then 0.5mg/kg q 5-10 min to max 3mg/kg. **Cardiac arrest:** use 100mg once. **Maintenance** 20-60 µg/kg/min (1-4mg/min). **Rebolus** 1mg/kg and increase infusion for breakthrough arrhythmias. Reduce infusion after 1 day. No need to taper before discontinuing. **Mix** 1 gram / 125 mL D5W = 8 mg/mL.

Renal failure: Minimal T½ change: no dose Δ, not dialyzed. GX accumulates (above)

Side-effects: Neurologic, may be due to MEGX. Mild: drowsiness, slurred speech, paresthesias, confusion; seen almost universally > 7 µg/mL. Severe: seizures.

Interactions: Half-life prolonged by beta-blockers (which decrease hepatic blood flow) and by cimetidine (reduces hepatic metabolism).

Levels: Initial level (µg/mL) ≅ 0.1*dose(mg)/min. 2.3-6 µg/mL considered therapeutic but levels up to 6-9 µg/mL may be required. Seizures seen at levels > 5 µg/mL.

Magnesium

Action: Replacement; anticonvulsant esp. in preeclampsia, may suppress Torsades de Pointes, may improve outcome in acute MI. In severe ↓ Mg, deficit is 1-

[194] Flamenbaum & Dubrow, "Labetalol," in Messerli FH(ed.) Cardiovascular Drug Therapy, Philadelphia: Saunders, 1990.
[195] Cummins RO (ed.), American Heart Association, Textbook of Advanced Cardiac Life Support, Dallas: AHA, 1994, pp 7-6-7-8.

2mEq/kg; half of administered Mg is excreted renally. Replace half in first day and remainder in 2-3d. Serum levels correlate poorly with body stores. 1 g = 8.12 mEq.

<u>PO</u> absorption is ~50% unless malabsorption is etiology of low Mg. Magnesium hydroxide: MOM 5mL/400mg/20mEq/1tsp lid.

<u>IV:</u> **Replacement:** Mg Sulfate 6g/49mEq in 1 L D5W IV over 4hrs then q8hrs; or give 1-4g of 10% < 1.5mL/min. **Acute MI**[196]: 1g of 50% IV push over 5 min then 8 g in 50mL IV over 24 hrs. **Torsades:** 2-4 g IV rapid push. **Eclampsia:** 2-4g IV push over 2-4 min then 1-3mg/hr titrated to respiratory drive, loss of patellar reflexes, levels. Levels of 4-7 therapeutic in eclampsia & seizures. Levels>7 toxic.

<u>IM:</u> IV dose as 1-5g 25% solution q4-6hrs.

<u>Side effects:</u> hypotension, hypothermia, CNS depression, respiratory paralysis. Flushing and atropine-responsive bradycardia. Extreme caution in renal failure.

Mannitol[197]

<u>Action:</u> Osmotic diuretic used theoretically to preserve intravascular volume; to ↓ intracerebral pressure by dehydration; to ↓ intraocular pressure; and to remove toxins, eg IV contrast, salicylates, barbiturates, TCAs, lithium. 5% mannitol = 275 mOsm/L; 25% = 1375 mOsm/L.

<u>Kinetics:</u> Renal excretion 80% in 3 hr. V_d extracellular fluid 0.2 L/kg. Half-life ~ 100 min, longer in renal failure. Osmotic effect 15 min, diuresis hours, reduction of intracerebral/intraocular pressure 3-8 hrs.

<u>IV:</u> **Maximum** 6 g/kg/24 hr. **Toxin** 50-200 g daily as 5-25% to maintain urine output 100-500 mL/hr. **Cerebral edema** 1.5-2.0g/kg as 15-25% over 30-60 min; repeat q 6-12 hrs. **Diuretic** 50-100 g as 5-25% over 1-2 hr. Replace urine q 2-4 hrs prn. Consider 1-2 **test doses** 200 mg/kg over 3-5 min when treating oliguric renal failure & uncertain volume.

<u>Adverse effects:</u> Dehydration, electrolyte abnormalities, hematocrit fall through cell shrinkage; catastrophic **pulmonary edema** and volume overload may exacerbate renal failure. Rebound ↑ ICP sometimes seen ~12 hrs after infusion if mannitol crosses blood-brain barrier.

Methylene Blue[198]

<u>Action:</u> Reduces methemoglobin ferric → ferrous state: NADPH-dehydrogenase reduces methylene blue which then reduces methemoglobin. Requires NADPH generated by pentose phosphate pathway, itself requiring G-6-PD.

<u>Indication:</u> Symptomatic methemoglobinemia > 40%. Note: remove toxins as warranted by charcoal lavage, catharsis, hemodialysis. Exchange transfusion or hemodialysis if > 70% MetHb.

<u>Contraindication:</u> G-6-PD deficiency, induces hemolysis (note alternative ascorbic acid has very slow onset).

<u>IV:</u> 1-2 mg/kg of 1% solution, repeat in 1 hour if cyanosis persists.

<u>Adverse reactions:</u> Colors urine bright blue-green. Irritates bladder. Cumulative doses > 7mg/kg can cause dyspnea, chest pain, tremor, cyanosis, hemolysis.

Metoprolol

<u>Action & Kinetics & Warnings:</u> See beta-blockers on page 98.

<u>Kinetics:</u> T½ 3-7hrs. Liver elimination. No dose Δ in renal failure. Onset 30-60min po.

---

[196] Benefit in MI shown in a single-center randomized trial (Woods KL, et al, "Intravenous magnesium sulphate in suspected acute myocardial infarction: results of the second Leicester Intravenous Magnesium Intervention Trial (LIMIT-2)," Lancet, 1992;339(8809):1553-8.) not substantiated in a larger randomized trial (ISIS-4, Lancet, 1995;345:669-85); Note ISIS-4 administered Mg after fibrinolytic therapy, conceivably after therapeutic window.
[197] American Medical Association, Drug Evaluations, 6/e, Chicago: AMA Publications, 1986. IM Weiner & GH Mudge, "Diuretics" in Goodman & Gilman, Pharmacological Basis of Therapeutics, 7/e, NY:Macmillan, 1985.
[198] ER Jaffe, "Methaemoglobinemia," Clin Haematol, 1981;10(1):99; A Mansouri, "Review: methemoglobinemia," Am J Med Sci, 1985;289(5):200.

IV: **MI:** 5mg IV q 2 minutes x 3 as tolerated. If 15mg tolerated, give 50mg po q6hrs x 48hrs then 100 bid. Begin po 15 min after last IV dose.

PO: **Angina, HTN:** 100-400mg/d. Maximal effect over one week.

Midazolam[199] *(Versed)*

Action: Benzodiazepine activates GABA. receptor promoting CNS depression. Amnestic, anxiolytic, muscle relaxant used as sedative and anticonvulsant.

Kinetics: Liver metabolism, renal excretion. Onset 3-5 min, T½ 2-6hr.

IV: 0.01-0.05 mg/kg IV over 2 min or 0.05-0.2 mg/kg IM, observe for 2 minutes before rebolusing; > 5 mg usually unnecessary. **Elderly** pts use 0.25-0.5 mg as initial dose. **Maintenance** 25% of dose required for induction. **Dose must be individualized & titrated. Oximetric monitoring recommended.**

Renal failure: T½ unchanged, distribution different. Use 50% for GFR<10.

Contraindications: Narrow-angle glaucoma.

Adverse reactions: Respiratory depression, hypotension.

Pregnancy: Teratogenic.

Milrinone *(Primacor)*

Action: Inotrope-vasodilator, phosphodiesterase-III inhibitor used in CHF.

IV: Load 50 µg/kg over 10 min, then 0.375 (minimum), 0.500 (standard), or 0.750 µ g/kg/min infusion typically for less than 72 hrs. Mix: Add 80 mL to 20mg/20mL vial to make 200 µg/mL.

Kinetics: Onset 5-15 min. Terminal elimination T½ 2.3 hr. 70% protein-bound, 80% urine elimination, remainder glucuronide.

Renal Failure: 40% dose for GFR<5; 60% dose for GFR≈30.

Interactions: Precipitates IV furosemide.

Side Effects: Hypotension, tachycardia, aggravates ventricular arrhythmia, accelerates ventricular response to atrial fibrillation. Headache. Contains bisulfite.

Naloxone[200] *(Narcan)*

Action: Direct opiate competitive antagonist, no agonist properties.

Kinetics: T½30-80 minutes in adults. IM more prolonged than IV. Liver metabolism.

Indication: Opiate overdose, reversal of opiate sedation/hypotension.

IV/IM/SQ: 0.1-0.2mg (0.4mg/mL) IV q2-3 min to total 10mg, then question opiate intoxication. Postop 0.1-0.2 IV q2-3min. Mix 2mg/250mL=0.008 mg/mL; 50mL/hr=0.4mg/hr. Give 0.4-0.8 mg/h titrated to effect, or give 2/3 dose that caused reversal hourly.

Caution: Abrupt reversal of narcotic depression can cause HTN, tachy, N/V, tremulousness, seizures (especially with normeperidine), arrest. Rare postop experience of hypotension, VF, VT but associated with cardiac drugs. Incompatible with polyanions (heparin, albumin), alkali, bisulfite. Narcotic half-life may exceed naloxone's. Large doses needed for pentazocine or propoxyphene.

Neostigmine

See "Anticholinesterases" on page 97.

Neuromuscular blockers:
Succinylcholine, Pancuronium, Atracurium, Vecuronium

Warning: **In patients not already intubated, neuromuscular blockers should be used only by physicians skilled in advanced airway management including endotracheal intubation.**

Action: Quaternary ammonium compounds, nicotinic cholinergic blockers which ↓

---

[199] Shapiro BA, *et al*, "Practice parameters for intravenous analgesia and sedation for adult patients in the intensive care unit: an executive summary. Society of Critical Care Medicine," Crit Care Med, 1995;23(9):1596-600.
[200] RS Wassman "Naloxone," in Goldfrank's Toxicologic Emergencies, 4/e (1990), pp 444-5.

motor response at neuromuscular junction. <u>Nondepolarizing agents</u> (pancuronium, atracurium, vecuronium) block ACh action without altering resting electrical potential. <u>Depolarizing agents</u> (succinylcholine) phase I: tetany and twitching from depolarization, electrolyte shifts; phase II: resembles nondepolarizing block. Affects sequentially: eyes, face, neck THEN limbs, abdomen, chest THEN diaphragm.

<u>Side-effects:</u>

<u>Histamine release:</u> succinylcholine > atracurium > pancuronium + gallamine > vecuronium. <u>Cardiovascular:</u> Hypotension, bronchospasm, conduction abnormality. Seen in all nondepolarizing agents except atracurium & vecuronium. <u>Crosses placenta.</u> <u>Malignant hyperthermia:</u> Treat with dantrolene (see page 101) ± procainamide. <u>Muscarinic</u> side effects: bradycardia, hypotension, salivation.

<u>Reversal:</u> Nondepolarizing agents with cholinesterase inhibitors (neostigmine, pyridostigmine, edrophonium) + atropine; IV Calcium.

<u>Caution/Interactions:</u> Hyperkalemia especially with digitalis & succ (causes release of cellular K), Myasthenia gravis, myasthenic syndromes, hypothyroidism, dehydration, aminoglycosides. Potentiated by hypokalemia, hypocalcemia, hypermagnesemia, respiratory acidosis, metabolic alkalosis, hypothermia, liver failure. Prolonged infusion: little data; prolonged neuromuscular blockade has been demonstrated in many pts on vecuronium > 2 d, esp those with renal failure.[201]

Succinylcholine

<u>Dose:</u> 1-1.5mg/kg IV, onset 1 minute, duration 5-10 min. Rapidly hydrolyzed in plasma. No maintenance bolus; infusion 2.5-15 mg/min.

<u>Advantage:</u> Speedy onset; doesn't cross placenta. Kidney-independent.

<u>Disadvantages:</u> Depolarization causes hyperkalemia (usual increase 0.5 mM); avoid in predisposed pts, eg renal insufficiency, burns, crush injury. Prolonged paralysis with decreased hepatic production of cholinesterase. Vasopressor action may ↑ intracranial pressure. Avoid in stroke, 48 hrs-6 mo after head or spinal cord injury: proliferation of postjunctional receptors ⇒ denervation hypersensitivity. Bradyarrhythmias (rare in adults; prophylax with atropine).

Pancuronium:

<u>Dose:</u> 0.04-0.1mg/kg; for intubation 0.06-.16.mg/kg. Repeat 0.01 mg/kg q 25-60min. Half-life 2 hours with normal renal function.

<u>Disadvantage:</u> Contraindicated in renal failure, causes tachycardia, hypertension, salivation. Histamine release.

Vecuronium

<u>Dose:</u> 0.07-0.10 mg/kg IV for intubation 2-3 minutes, 25% recovery in 25-30 minutes. Reduce to 0.04-0.06 if used after succinylcholine. Maintenance 0.010-0.015 mg/kg q 25-40 minutes. Infusion 1μg/kg/min; mix 50mg/250mL = 200μ g/mL. T½ 65-75 minutes.

<u>Advantages:</u> No adjustment for renal failure; no adverse hemodynamic effects; no histamine release; no cumulative effects on duration of blockade from excessive dosing.

Atracurium

<u>Dose:</u> 0.4-0.5 mg/kg (0.3-0.4 after succ), maintenance 0.08-0.1mg/kg. Intubation 2-2.5min, max action 3-5 min. Recovery 35-40 min. Continuous infusion 5-9μ g/kg/min.

<u>Advantages:</u> No adjustment for renal or liver failure. Hoffman elimination / ester hydrolysis.

<u>Disadvantages:</u> Histamine release.

---

[201] V Segredo, et al, "Persistent paralysis in critically ill patients after long-term administration of vecuronium," N Engl J Med, 1992;327(8):524-8.

Comparison summary of neuromuscular blockers				
	Succinylcholine	Pancuronium	Atracurium	Vecuronium
Intubating dose (mg/kg)	1.0-1.5	0.06-0.08	0.4-0.5	0.07-0.1
Maintenance bolus (mg/kg)	—	0.01-0.015	0.08-0.1	0.01-0.015
Infusion	2.5-15 mg/min		5-9μg/kg/min	~1μg/kg/min
Intubate time	60s	2-3 min	2-2.5 min	2.4 min
Time to recover 25% twitch	5-10 min	60-90 min	30-45 min	25-30 min
Elimination route	Plasma pseudo cholinesterase	60-80% renal; rest hepatic	Hoffman ester hydrolysis	10-20% renal; 80-90% liver
Renal failure[a]	No	No	Yes	Yes
Liver failure[a]	Yes	No	Yes	No
Histamine release	Yes	Yes	Yes	No

a: May be used without dosage adjustment in these conditions

Nicardipine IV *(Cardene)*

Action: Dihydropyridine calcium-channel blocker relaxes vascular >> cardiac smooth muscle. Used as parenteral hypotensive as alternative to nitroprusside.
Kinetics: α-T½ 2.7 min, β-T½ 45 min, γ-T½ 14hr. Rapid hepatic clearance.
IV: Mix 25 mg ampule in 240 mL fluid = 0.1 mg/mL. Infuse 5.0 mg/hr (50mL/hr), titrate additional 2.5 mg/hr q 5-15 min until desired BP or maximum 15.0 mg/hr. After reaching BP goal, reduce infusion to 3.0 mg/hr. BP falls ~50% after 30±7 min after discontinuation. **Transition to oral:** Give po nicardipine 1 hr before discontinuing infusion.
PO: 20 mg q 8 ≈ 0.5 mg/hr; 30 mg q 8 ≈ 1.2 mg/hr; 40 mg q 8 ≈ 2.2 mg/hr.
Renal failure: Delayed clearance.
Liver failure: Delayed clearance. May exacerbate portal hypertension.
Contraindication: Vasodilators contraindicated in critical aortic stenosis.
Caution: Causes reflex tachycardia which may provoke/exacerbate myocardial ischemia. Negative inotrope in severe LV dysfunction. Decreases GFR in renal dysfunction. No antiadrenergic effects to warrant use in pheochromocytoma, β-blocker withdrawal, *etc.*
Interactions: Levels increased by cimetidine. Increases cyclosporine levels.
Pregnancy: Class C. Embryocidal in certain animals.

Nitrite

See "Overdose" under the "Nitroprusside" section on page 113.

Nitroglycerin

Action: Dose-dependent arterial and venous vasodilator. ↑s coronary perfusion, decreases MVO₂, PCWP, PVR, SVR. Reduces infarct extent in acute MI. Combined with dobutamine in ischemic CHF.
Kinetics: Plasma half-life 1-4 min.
IV: Mix 25 mg in 250 mL D5 or NS = 100μg/mL. **Note** absorbed by plastic/polyvinyl chloride. Begin 5-10μg/min (3mL/hr), titrate 10-20 μg/min increments q 3-5min. Predominant hypotensive above 200 μg/min. For PVC tubing, start at 25μg/min.
3% Ointment: Antianginal onset 30 min. Begin 1.5inch q4. **Explosive** during cardioversion.
Renal failure: Half-life unchanged. No dosage adjustment.
Contraindication: Increased intracranial pressure, narrow-angle glaucoma, ↓ed cerebral perfusion, constrictive pericarditis, pericardial tamponade.
Caution: IV reduces preload in RV infarcts.
Side effects: Headache, N/V/abd discomfort, dizziness, dermatitis.

Nitroprusside *(Nipride)*

Action: Arterial & venous vasodilator. Free nitroso group (NO) inhibits excitation-contraction coupling of vascular, not visceral, smooth muscle. Reacts with Hb to yield met-Hb & unstable compound releasing cyanide. CN converted (using thiosulfate) in liver and kidney to thiocyanate. May shunt blood away from renal/splanchnic bed and from diseased coronary arteries. T½ < 10 min. Used for afterload reduction in acute CHF, MR, AI, VSD. Reduces for all causes of severe HTN including pheochromocytoma. Second-line agent in eclampsia.

IV: Mix 50mg in 250mL D5W = 200µg/mL. Range 0.5-10µg/kg/min. Titrate in 10mg/min increments q 3-15 min. **Withdraw slowly** to avoid rebound vasoconstriction.

Renal failure: Half-time unchanged. No dosage adjustment. Thiocyanate accumulates; It can be dialyzed.

Levels: Blood **cyanide** levels not predictive of tissue levels or of toxicity. Follow **thiocyanate** daily after 24-48 hr infusion, especially if abnormal CNS baseline. Symptoms @ 60 µg/mL; "toxicity" @ 100 µg/mL. No problems usually when infused < 72hrs at less than 3 µg/kg/min (normal kidneys) or less than 1 µ g/kg/min (anuric). Thiocyanate elimination T½ 3d (normals), 9d (renal dysfunction). Keep **methemoglobin** < 10%.

Toxicity: Manifested clinically by tinnitus, blurred vision, confusion, psychosis, seizure, delirium, lactic acidosis, marrow depression, pink color, electromechanical dissociation. **Failure to respond** to adequate infusion or **metabolic acidosis** may represent increased free cyanide. Infusion of **hydroxycobalamin** (not cyanocobalamin) 25 mg/hr may reduce cyanide toxicity. **Cyanide** accumulates in liver disease; **thiocyanate** accumulates in renal dysfunction.

Contraindications: Severe liver disease (rhodanase deficiency), vitamin B12 deficiency, hypothyroidism (exacerbated by thiocyanate), aortic dissection, AS, aortic coarctation, Leber congenital optic atrophy or tobacco amblyopia (absent rhodanase).

Caution: Hypovolemia, renal disease, cerebrovascular disease.

Overdose: (1) Amyl nitrite 15-30sec/min until sodium nitrite available. (2) 3% sodium nitrite 2.5-5mL/min up to 10-15mL, may repeat 50% dose if signs return. (3) Sodium thiosulfate 12.5g/50mL D5 IV over 10min. (4) Thiocyanate removed by hemodialysis.

Pregnancy: Class C; considered 2nd-line in preeclampsia after hydralazine & labetalol.

Norepinephrine *(Levophed)*

Action: Potent β-1 and α-agonist. No β-2 action (unlike epi). β-1 prominent at low doses; α-1 predominates at higher doses. Vasoconstriction causes ↑ afterload & M_vO_2 ↓ splanchnic perfusion, exacerbates peripheral ischemia, but spares cerebral and coronary circulation which have fewer α-adrenergic receptors. Baroreceptor stimulation causes net balanced HR and CO. Arrhythmogenic, but less than epi. Chronic use → decreased circulatory volume related to vasoconstriction. Often used concurrently with low-dose dopamine. Compared with epi: half as potent chronotrope and inotrope, equipotent vasoconstrictor, no vasodilator properties.

Indications: (1) Cardiogenic shock unresponsive to DA, DBA, IABP. (2) Cardiogenic shock or EMD secondary to pulmonary embolism.

IV: **Mix** 4,6,8mg/250mL D5W (not NS) = 16,32,64 µg/mL. Initial 1µg/min, max 40µ g/min. Incompatible with alkali.

Cautions: Avoid extravasation; use long IV or central lines. Peripheral a-lines may be artifactually damped by vasoconstriction. Suspect volume depletion with hypotension, esp. with chronic use. Correct hypocalcemia to preserve contractility. Correct volume first.

Extravasation: See phentolamine page 117.

Contraindications: MAOI or TCA ⇒ hypertension.

NSAIDS[202]

Name	Starting dose (mg)	Max / d	cox2 / cox1[c]	T½ hr
Salicylates				
Aspirin	650-1300 q4-6h	a	155	4-15
Choline Mg trisalicylate (Trilisate)	750-1500 bid	a		4-15
Salsalate (Disalcid)	1000 bid-1500 tid	a		4-15
Acetic or Carboxylic Acids				
Diclofenac (Voltaren)	50-75 bid	200	0.7	2
Diflunisal (Dolobid)	250 bid	1500		7-15
Etodolac (Lodine)	200 tid-qid	1200		2-7
Indomethacin (Indocin)	25 tid-qid	200	60	3-11
Ketorolac (Toradol)	60[b] mg then 30 mg q 6 hr IM or 15-60 then 30 q 6hr IV or 10-20 mg po q 6 hr	120; max 5d		5-12
Nabumetone (Relafen)	1000-2000 qd	2000	0.014	2.5-4
Sulindac (Clinoril)	150-200 bid	400	100	16
Tolmetin (Tolectin)	400 tid	2000		1-2
Propionic Acids				
Fenoprofen (Nalfon)	300-600 qid	3200		2
Flurbiprofen (Ansaid)	50-100 tid	300		3-4
Ibuprofen (Motrin)	400 qid	3200		2
Ketoprofen (Orudis)	75 tid	300		2
Naproxen (Naprosyn)	250-500 bid	1000	0.59	13
Naproxen sodium (Anaprox)	275 q6-8h	1375	0.59	
Oxaprozin (Daypro)	Load 1200 then 600-1800 qd	1800		20-40
Fenamic Acids				
Meclofenamate (Meclomen)	50 tid-qid	400		2-3
Mefenamic acid (Ponstel)	250 qid	1000		
Enolic acids				
Phenylbutazone (Butazolidin)	100 tid	600		40-80
Piroxicam (Feldene)	20 qd	20	600	30-86

a Maximum salicylate dose determined by symptoms & blood level
b Comparable to morphine 12 mg.
c Ratio of IC_{50} of cyclooxygenase-2/cox-1; higher ratio suggest greater GI toxicity[203]

Octreotide (Sandostatin)

Action: Synthetic somatostatin analogue suppresses serotonin and GI peptides gastrin, vasoactive intestinal peptide, insulin, glucagon, secretin, motilin, amylase, lipase, growth hormone, TSH. Also decreases splanchnic blood flow. Used for symptomatic VIPomas & carcinoids, intractable diarrhea as in AIDS & fistulae, control of variceal esophagus hemorrhage, acromegaly.
Kinetics: T½ 0.2-1.4hr. Hepatic metabolism & renal excretion.
IV: **Variceal esophagus hemorrhage:** 50 µg bolus (1 mL over 3 min) then 50 µg/hr × 48 hr (mix 1200 µg in 250 mL D5W infuse @ 10mL/hr)[204].
SQ: **Other:** Begin 50 µg SQ qd, advance prn up to 350 µg bid. Monitor glucose,

[202] Brooks PM, Day RO, "Nonsteroidal antiinflammatory drugs--differences and similarities," N Engl J Med,1991;324(24):1716-25.
[203] Hayllar J, Bjarnason I, "NSAIDS, Cox-2 inhibitors, and the gut," Lancet 1995; 346(8974):521-2.
[204] JJY Sung, et al, "Octreotide infusion or emergency sclerotherapy for variceal haemorrhage," Lancet 1993; 342:637-41.

urinary 5-HIAA, VIP
<u>Interactions</u>: Inactivated by TPN solution. Reduces insulin requirements.
<u>Adverse effects</u>: Biliary sludge & stones. Pain at injection site. N/V/abd pain.

Opiate analgesics[205]

	Oral:Parenteral equivalence	Duration (hrs)	Equipotent dose parenteral (mg)[a]
Morphine	6:1	4-5	1.0
Morphine-SR (MS-Contin)	—	8-12	3.0
Buprenorphine[c] (Buprenex)	—	4-6	0.3
Butorphanol[c] (Stadol)	—	4-6	0.2
Codeine	3:2	4-6	13
Fentanyl[206] (Sublimaze)	—	1-2	0.01
Hydromorphone (Dilaudid)	5:1	4-5	0.13
Levorphanol (LevoDromoran)	2:1	4-6	0.2
Meperidine (Demerol)[b]	4:1	3-5	7.5
Methadone (Dolophine)	2:1	4-6	1.0
Nalbuphine[c] (Nubain)	—	4-6	1.0
Oxycodone (Percodan)	—	4-5	1.0
Pentazocine[c] (Talwin)	5:1	4-6	3.0
Propoxyphene (Darvon)	—	4-6	6.5

a Potency relative to morphine: *eg* 0.01 mg fentanyl ~ 1 mg morphine.
b Avoid meperidine in renal failure, since normeperidine (chief metabolite) accumulates and may cause seizures.
c Agonist-antagonist narcotic

Adjunctive analgesics[207]

	Dose range	Route	Use
NSAIDS			See NSAIDS (page 114).
Corticosteroids			
Dexamethasone	16-96 mg/d	PO/IV	Brain metastases & epidural spinal. cord compression
Prednisone	40-80 mg/d	PO	
Anticonvulants			
Carbamazepine	200-1600mg/d	PO	Neuropathic pain
Phenytoin	300-500 mg/d	PO	
Antidepressants			
Amitryptiline	25-150 mg/d	PO	Neuropathic pain
Doxepin	25-150 mg/d	PO	
Imipramine	20-100 mg/d	PO	
Trazodone	75-225 mg/d	PO	
Neuroleptics			
Methotrimeprazine	40-80 mg/d	IM	Analgesia, sedation, antiemetic
Antihistamines			
Hydroxyzine	300-450 mg/d	IM	Enhance postop opiate analgesia; also ↓ anxiety, insomnia, & nausea

205 Goodman & Gilman's The pharmacolgical basis of therapeutics, 9/e, 1996, New York: McGraw-Hill, p 535. A Jacox, *et al*, "New clinical-practice guidelines for the management of pain in patients with cancer," N Engl J Med 1994; 330(9):651-5.
206 Shapiro BA, *et al*, "Practice parameters for intravenous analgesia and sedation for adult patients in the intensive care unit: an executive summary. Society of Critical Care Medicine," Crit Care Med, 1995;23(9):1596-600.
207 A Jacox, *et al*, "New clinical-practice guidelines for the management of pain in patients with cancer," N Engl J Med 1994; 330(9):651-5

	Dose range	Route	Use
Anxiolytics			
Lorazepam	0.5-2+ mg tid	PO	
Diazepam	2.5-10 qid	PO	
Muscle Relaxants			
Cyclobenzaprine	10-30 mg tid	PO	Relieve musculoskeletal spasm
Local anesthetics			
Lidocaine	5 mg/kg/d	IV/SQ	Neuropathic pain
Mexiletine	450-600 mg/d	PO	
Tocainide	20 mg/d	PO	
Psychostimulants			
Dextroamphetamine	5-10 mg/d	PO	Enhance opioids, ↓ sedation
Methylphenidate	10-15 mg/d	PO	

Pancuronium
See "Neuromuscular blockers" on page 111.

Pentobarbital *(Nembutal)*
Action: Barbiturate used in generalized anesthesia and in treatment of generalized convulsive status epilepticus. Patients should be intubated with continuous EKG and intraarterial BP monitoring. Plasma T½ 15-50h.
IV: Load 15 mg/kg over 60 min, then 0.5 mg/kg/hr to achieve burst-suppression pattern on EEG. Follow level (range 15-40 µg/mL)
Renal failure: Unchanged. No dosage adjustment. Not dialyzed.
Side effects: Profound hypotension, respiratory depression. Direct myocardial suppressant. Patients often require vasopressor/inotropic support when using this agent.

Phenobarbital
Action: Barbiturate used in generalized and partial seizures.
Kinetics: Oral absorption 70-90%, peak 8-12 h, brain 10-15h. Elimination 25% renal unchanged, 75% liver metabolites as urine. T½ 2-6 d.
PO: 100-300 mg/day (1-5mg/kg/d), therapeutic levels after 2-3 weeks.
IV: 20mg/kg load at 50-100 (ideal <60) mg/minute. Note peak onset 30 minutes; therefore do not administer continuously until seizures stop.
Levels 10-25 µg/mL therapeutic, 10-40 acute therapy, 50 coma.
Renal failure: T½ 5-7d. For GFR>50 give q8-12h; GFR 10-50: q8-12h; GFR<10: q12-16h. Supplement full dose after hemodialysis/CAVH; ½ dose after CAPD.
Side effects: Respiratory depression, hypotension. Sedation, nystagmus and ataxia at toxic levels. Agitation and confusion in elderly. Maculopapular, morbilliform, scarlatiniform rashes 1-3%; erythema multiforme or Stevens-Johnson syndrome rarely. Chronic: megaloblastic anemia responsive to folate, osteomalacia responsive to Vitamin D.
Drug interactions: Induces hepatic microsome oxidase. Decreases levels of phenytoin, warfarin, beta blockers, corticosteroids, contraceptives, quinidine, doxycycline, vitamin D. Increases levels of TCAs. Displaces thyroxine from albumin. Causes production of toxic metabolites of chlorocarbon anesthetics & carbon tetrachloride.

Phentolamine *(Regitine)*
Action: Nonspecific α-adrenergic antagonist used in excess adrenergic states, eg, pheochromocytoma, clonidine withdrawal, MAO inhibitors interfering with breakdown of norepinephrine, cocaine toxicity. Also used to limit skin necrosis from extravasation of catecholamines.
Kinetics: Liver metabolism. Plasma half-life 19 min.
Extravasation of catecholamines: Infiltrate area liberally 5-10mg/10-15mL via 25g needle. Conspicuous hyperemia if used within 12hrs.

<u>IV:</u> **Pheochromocytoma:** 5mg IV/IM given 1-2 hrs preoperatively, titrate for effect. Administering β-blocker before α-blocker may cause severe unopposed α-mediated vasocontriction; always give α-blocker first.
<u>Counteract:</u> With fluids, norepinephrine, **not** epinephrine.

Phenylephrine *(Neo-Synephrine)*

<u>Action:</u> Postsynaptic alpha adrenergic agonist with virtually no beta activity. Vasoconstrictor as potent as norepinephrine but almost entirely without the chronotropic and inotropic activity. Causes marked reflex **bradycardia** that can be blocked by atropine. Used for hypotension, shock, spinal anesthesia, drug-related hypotension. Less arrhythmogenic than other catecholamines. Good anesthesia pressor in combination with cardiac irritants like cyclopropane or halothane. Unlike methoxamine, constricts coronary, cerebral, pulmonary vessels.
<u>Dose:</u> 0.1-0.5mg IV q 15 minutes. Mix 10mg in 250mL fluid. Start infusion at 100-180 μg/min. Titrate down to maintenance dose, usually 40-60μg/min. Maximum infusion rate not specified by manufacturer; they recommend adding additional 10mg increments to infusion bag to maintain acceptable infusion rate.
<u>Caution:</u> MAO inhibitors, TCAs, & oxytocic agents potentiate the pressor effect, use vastly reduced doses of phenylephrine.

Phenytoin *(Dilantin)*

<u>Indications:</u> Generalized, partial complex, simple partial seizures. <u>Not</u> used in absence, myoclonic, atonic seizures. Used also for arrhythmias of digitalis toxicity & after Tetralogy repair. <u>Enhances</u> AV node conduction. T½ 24 hrs.
<u>PO</u> Load 400mg, then 300mg q2hrs x 2. Then 100 tid next day. Or begin 100 tid. Once stable may switch to once-daily if no adverse Sx. Increase doses in increments of 50mg. Steady-state levels 7-10d after dose Δ.
<u>IV</u> Load 18-20mg/kg not faster than 50mg/min, followed by maintenance 100mg IV q6-8. Observe for ↓ BP & arrhythmia, especially rapid infusion. **Fosphenytoin**, a water-soluble prodrug, causes less hypotension, is dispensed in phenytoin-equivalents, can be administered up to 150 mg/min IV.
<u>Levels:</u> Therapeutic 10-20μg/mL, may use up to 30-40 μg/mL in comatose pt with status epilepticus. Obtain 2 hrs after IV load. **Free phenytoin levels** (therapeutic 1-2μg/mL) increased by renal failure, albumin<2.8, liver failure, warfarin, sulfonamides, salicylates, valproate.
<u>Dose adjustments:</u> Based on levels, 0.5-1.0 mg/kg/day for "medical" or prophylactic treatment; 1.5-2mg/kd/day if severe brain disease.
<u>Renal failure:</u> T½ unchanged. No adjustment. See "levels" above.
<u>Side effects:</u> Hypotension given IV (mixed in propylene glycol); Folate antagonism (megaloblastic anemia), vitamin K antagonism, vitamin D antagonism (institutionalized pts), inhibition of insulin secretion, interstitial nephritis. <u>Toxicity:</u> Ataxia, diplopia, slurred speech, stupor. <u>Hypersensitivity:</u> Fever, lymphadenopathy, eosinophilia, blood dyscrasias, polyarteritis, Stevens-Johnson. <u>Chronic:</u> Gingival hyperplasia, hirsutism, coarsening of facial features, sensory polyneuropathy, cerebellar degeneration, pseudolymphoma.
<u>Interactions:</u> **Decrease phenytoin levels:** carbamazepine, sucralfate, chronic EtOH, calcium antacids, folic acid, reserpine. **Increase phenytoin levels:** Amiodarone, Chloramphenicol, chlordiazepoxide, cimetidine, diazepam, disulfiram, estrogens, isoniazid, phenothiazines, salicylates, sulfonamides, trimethoprim, trazodone. **Free phenytoin** increased in hyperbilirubinemia, hypoalbuminemia, uremia. **Idiosyncratic effect:** Phenobarbital, valproate. Tricyclics lower seizure threshold. **Action altered by phenytoin:** Corticosteroids, increases metabolism of warfarin, doxycycline, estrogens, primidone, quinidine, rifampin, theophylline, vitamin D.
<u>Pregnancy:</u> Extensive experience, fetal hydantoin syndrome, neonatal coagulopathy, short-term use probably safe.

Phosphorus[208]

PO: 1-2 g daily in 3 divided doses, increment as tolerated. Milk (skim 1 L = 1 g P).
Neutra-Phos 4×1250 mg tabs = 1 g P + 28.5mEq Na + 28.5mEq K; Neutra-Phos-K 4×1450 mg tabs = 1 g P + 57mEq K.

IV: Reserve for pts who are symptomatic or unable to tolerate po. Dispensed 94mg = 3 mMol phosphorus + 4.4 mEq Na or K per mL. Traditional 0.08-0.2mmol/kg in 50-500mL fluid over 6 hrs. Or administer the following in maintenance fluids or in q 12 hr boluses infused over 6 hrs. Guide subsequent doses by serum levels.

Serum P (mg/dl)	Initial IV dose (mmol/kg IBW/day)	
	Uncomplicated	Symptoms, chronic, or multifactorial
1.6-2.1	0.15	0.15-0.3
1.2-1.5	0.15-0.3	0.3
0.8-1.1	0.3	0.3-0.45
< 0.8	0.45-0.6	0.6

Side effects: hypocalcemic tetany (also if given too rapidly), tissue calcification, hyperkalemia, diarrhea if given po too rapidly.

Interactions: Precipitates in fluids with calcium gluconate > 9.6 mEq/l.

Physostigmine

See "Anticholinesterases" on page 97.

Pilocarpine

Action: Direct-acting parasympathomimetic. Used in acute angle-closure glaucoma. Miosis begins in 10-30 min, persists 4-8hrs. Intraocular pressure reduces in 60 min, maximum 75 min, persists 4-14hrs.

Dose: For emergency angle closure glaucoma: 1 drop of 2% solution in affected eye q 5-10 min for 3-6 doses then q 1-3 hrs until IOP controlled. To prevent bilateral attack, some instill 1 drop 1-2% solution to unaffected eye q 6-8hrs. If IOP inadequately controlled, consider systemic acetazolamide & mannitol.

Caution: Systemic cholinergic; systemic absorption ↑ in corneal abrasion.

Pralidoxime (2-PAM)[209]

Action: Reactivates acetylcholinesterase rendered inactive by organophosphate insecticides. Quaternary ammonium removes phosphoryl group from active enzyme site by nucleophilic attack, restoring cholinesterase activity. Also directly detoxifies certain organophosphates. Used to reverse (respiratory) muscle paralysis. Possible role in reverse overdose of carbamate anticholinesterase drugs (eg ambenonium, neostigmine, pyridostigmine) but less effective and controversial[210]. Possible role in tetanus therapy. Effectively reverses nicotinic toxicity (skeletal muscle & sympathetic ganglia); less effective against muscarinic effects but synergistic with atropine. Most effective given within 48hrs of exposure, indicated in all symptomatic exposures and those with RBC cholinesterase < 50% normal.

Kinetics: Onset 5-15 min IV, T½ 1-3 hrs. Renal excretion.

IV: 1-2 g (adult) 20-40 mg/kg (child). Give with atropine 2-6 mg. Reduce for renal insufficiency. Mix: Pulmonary edema: 50 mg/mL, administer > 5 min; otherwise 1-2g in 150 mL NS over 30 min. Repeat in 1 hr if muscle weakness continues or give 500 mg/hr. Repeat q 6-12 hrs for 24-48 hrs. Carbamate anticholinesterase toxicity: after atropine as above, 1-2 g IV then 250 mg IV q 5

[208] Desai TK, et al, "Hypocalcemia and hypophosphatemia in acutely ill patients," Crit Care Clin, 1987;3(4):927-41. Solomon SM; Kirby DF, "The refeeding syndrome: a review," JPEN, 1990;14(1):90-7.
[209] CK Aaron et al, "Insecticides: organophosphates & carbamates," in Goldfrank's Toxicologic Emergencies, 4/e (1990), pp 675-691.
[210] Kurtz PH, "Pralidoxime in the treatment of carbamate intoxication," Am J Emerg Med, 1990;8(1):68-70.
Lifshitz M, et al, "Carbamate poisoning and oxime treatment in children," Pediatrics, 1994;93(4):652-5.

min until reversal.
Caution: May precipitate myasthenic crisis. Reduce in renal failure.
Interactions: Theophylline, aminophylline, succinylcholine, respiratory depressants.
Adverse effects: Rapid infusion ⇒ tachycardia, laryngospasm, transient neuromuscular blockade, hypertension. Adverse effects difficult to distinguish from organophosphate toxicity.

Procainamide
Action: Class IA antiarrhythmic. Depresses conduction velocity & automaticity, prolongs refractoriness of atrial, ventricular myocardium and of accessory pathways while shortening refractoriness (via anticholinergic activity) of AV node. Mild anticholinergic without α-adrenergic blockade of quinidine. Negative inotropy in severe CHF. Prolongs P-R and Q-T intervals.
Metabolism: Acetylated to NAPA in liver (20% dose in slow and 30% dose in fast-acetylators. NAPA excreted in urine, accumulates in renal failure. PCA associated with lupus-like syndrome (like other aromatic amines, hydralazine and INH); infrequent in rapid-acetylators, in whom PCA levels are lower. NAPA not an aromatic amine. Plasma t ½ 3-5 hrs.
IV: **Load** 17 mg/kg (in 50mL D5W) at 1mL/min=20mg/min until arrhythmia stops, QRS is prolonged 50%, QT prolonged > 35%, hypotension (BP drops > 15%) ensues. **Maintenance** mix 1g in 100 mL D5W at 12 mL/hr = 2 mg/min. Range 2-8 mg/min (20-80 µg/kg/min).
PO/IM: Total 2-6g/day, begin at 50mg/kg/day. First dose one renal half-time (3-4 hrs) since last IV dose. Regular formulation q3-4hrs; SR q6hrs in equivalent total dose. If GFR =10-50 mL/min, give q6-12. If GFR<10mL/min give q8-24hrs, following levels. Peak PO levels 90 min.
Levels: PCA 4-10µg/mL, sometimes higher. NAPA 10-30 µg/mL.
Renal failure: Proc T½ 5-6 hrs; NAPA T½ 42-70h (normal 6-8h). Adjust for GFR>50: double interval; GFR 10-50: triple interval; GFR<10 quadruple interval. Supplement ½ dose after hemodialysis.
Contraindications: Complete AV block (⇒ asystole). SLE. Torsades. Long QT.
Caution: Myasthenia gravis, renal insufficiency, a-fib/flutter (may accelerate ventricular response), negative inotrope in high-doses (esp. severe LV dysfunction), prolongs SNRT in sick-sinus syndrome, unpredictable effects in digitalis toxicity, prolongs QT/Torsades. Note agranulocytosis and SLE syndromes. Peripheral vasodilator at supratherapeutic concentrations, especially during IV load.

Propofol[211] (Diprivan)
Action: Water-insoluble sedative-hypnotic causes rapid unconsciousness (crosses blood-brain barrier rapidly) and has short duration of action (rapid CNS redistribution & elimination). Formulated as lipid emulsion.
Kinetics: V_d=60L/kg reflects water-insolubility and extensive tissue redistribution. Plasma T½=5 min after 1hr infusion, 7 min after 10hr infusion. Eliminated by hepatic conjugation then renal excretion.
IV: **Infusion** 0.3mg/kg/h × 5 min then increment 0.3-0.6mg/kg/h q 5-10 min until desired sedation, max ~8mg/kg/h. Premixed 10mg/mL. If hypotension unlikely, consider initial **bolus** 1 mg/kg followed by 1-3mg/kg/h. Consider withdrawing sedation daily.
Renal failure: No apparent clinical effect.
Adverse effects: Dose-related myocardial depression, hypotension (often severe), respiratory depression/apnea and bradycardia. Pain at injection reduced with

---

[211] Shapiro BA, *et al*, "Practice parameters for intravenous analgesia and sedation for adult patients in the intensive care unit: an executive summary. Society of Critical Care Medicine," Crit Care Med, 1995;23(9):1596-600.

lidocaine or large vein. Lipid emulsion supports microbial overgrowth[212]; use sterile technique & replace drug/tubing q 12h.
Interactions: Concurrent opioids potentiate cardiopulmonary depression.

Propranolol (Inderal)

Action: Nonspecific β-adrenergic antagonist. See beta-blockers on page 98.
Kinetics: Liver metabolism, extensive first-pass. T½ 2-3 hrs IV; 3-6 hrs po.
Renal failure: T½ 1-6 hrs. No adjustments, not dialyzed.
IV: Bolus 0.5-1.0 mg q 5 min to effect; typical cumulative dose 0.075-0.15 mg/kg. Then rebolus 1 mg q 20-60 min or continuous 0.01-0.05 mg/min. End-point often resting or exertional bradycardia.
PO: 20-120 mg q6-8hrs. Sustained release 80-480 qd.
Contraindications & Warnings: See beta-blockers on page 98.
Interactions: Delays clearance of theophylline, lidocaine. Increases clearance of carbamazepine. Prolonged propranolol half-life from cimetidine. Shortened propranolol half-life from phenytoin, phenobarbital, carbamazepine. Antagonizes MAO inhibitors. Additive AV blocking with diltiazem, verapamil, digoxin.

Protamine

Action: Polycation from salmon sperm forms inactive complex with heparin, thereafter probably metabolized and fibrinolysed with release of some heparin. Weak anticoagulant effect via platelet and fibrinogen action. Neutralization instantly, note duration of protamine effect often shorter than heparin.
IV: 1 mg neutralizes ~ 100 units estimated circulating heparin, using estimated heparin T½ 60 min. Inject 10mg/mL over 1-3 min, not to exceed 50mg/10min. Excessive protamine probably causes mild anticoagulation.
Warning: Prior sensitization may occur from NPH insulin, protamine, vasectomy, predisposing to possible anaphylactoid rxns. Hyperheparinemia and bleeding may occur 0.5-18hrs after protamine administration. Too-rapid administration causes hypotension and anaphylactoid reaction. Incompatible with penicillins and cephalosporins.

Pyridostigmine

See "Anticholinesterases" on page 97.

Quinidine

Action: Class IA antiarrhythmic. Direct myocardial effects prolongs all intervals. Vagolytic activity increases conduction through SA and AV nodes. Alpha-adrenergic-antagonism causes vasodilatation, hypotension, reflex tachycardia most prominent after IV administration.
Kinetics: Bound to plasma proteins. Degraded by hepatic mixed-function oxidase. Not dialysable. T½ 6 h, prolonged in severe CHF, liver failure.
Equivalent doses

Salt	Dose	Quinidine Base	Bioavailable
Sulfate	200 mg	166 mg	166 mg
Gluconate	324 mg	200 mg	180 mg
Polygalacturonate	275 mg	166 mg	165 mg

Dose: 15mg/kg/d sulfate = 21 mg/kg/d gluconate q 6 hr or SR formulation q 8 hr.
Load: 200-300mg sulfate q 3-4hrs to total 1000-1200 mg has tolerable GI profile.
Renal failure: T½ 4-14 h. Use 50% dose GFR < 10. Supplement 100-200mg sulfate after hemodialysis, not CAPD.
Levels: 2-5 µg/mL therapeutic.
Side-effects: Torsades de points; conduction delay & bradycardia; diarrhea, N/V, HA, cinchonism.
Caution: Avoid low serum K, Ca, Mg. Attention to QT prolongation. Enhances

212 SN Bennet, *et al*, "Postoperative infections traced to contamination of an intravenous anesthetic, propofol," N Engl J Med 1995; 333(3):147-54.

hypotensive effect of other drugs; exacerbates QT prolongation from amiodarone & sotalol; neuromuscular blockade in myasthenia gravis; exacerbates sinus node dysfunction. QT_c prolongation exacerbated by LV dysfunction.[213]

Interactions: Digoxin levels double (decreased renal & nonrenal clearance & displacement from tissue binding sites, new steady-state > 5days). Higher quinidine levels: [cimetidine, verapamil (also additive α-blockade causes hypotension)]:inhibit hepatic metabolism; [acetazolamide & ? antacids]: alkalinize urine & increase renal reabsorption. Lower quinidine levels: [barbiturates, phenytoin, rifampin]: enhance liver metabolism; nifedipine esp. in LV dysfunction. Other: Warfarin effect occasionally enhanced.

Reteplase (rPA)

Action: Recombinant derivative of tissue plasminogen activator (tPA) with longer half-life, permits simplified dosing regimen with equivalent efficacy and side-effect profile. May be useful for prehospital thrombolysis.

Kinetics: Half-life 13-16 min, prolonged in renal and liver failure.

Contraindications, adverse reactions, reversal: See tPA (page 123).

IV: **Acute MI**[214]: 10 units IV bolus given twice, 30 minutes apart. Combine with aspirin and probably with heparin, as for tPA (page 123).

Streptokinase

Action: Converts plasminogen to plasmin which degrades fibrin clots. Purified from Group C streptococcus. Reduces mortality in acute MI. Used in hemodynamically unstable pulmonary emboli, and in acute arterial thromboembolism.

Kinetics: Half-life of activator complex is 23 min. Unknown metabolism; activator complex degraded in part by antistreptococcal antibodies. Hyperfibrinolytic effect lasts several hours; thrombin time and FDP elevated ~24 hrs. Loading dose required to overcome native antistreptococcal antibodies.

Contraindications: As for tissue plasminogen activator (see page 123). Also previous SK use. **Ineffective** given 5d-12mo of prior streptokinase or streptococcal infection.

IV: **Acute MI**: 1.5 million IU, of which 750,000 IU given over 10 min and remainder over 50 min. Give within 24hrs of pain onset; combine with aspirin, first tablet chewed; heparin not warranted[215]. **PE** (with hemodynamic compromise or involvement of ≥ an entire lobe): 250,000 IU over 30 min, then 100,000 IU over 24hrs (continue for 72 hrs if concurrent DVT).

Renal failure: No adjustment.

Adverse reactions: Hemorrhage (see contraindications), anaphylaxis, rash, fever, hypotension, reperfusion arrhythmias.

Reversal for hemorrhage: FFP, cryoprecipitate, ε-aminocaproic acid.

Succinylcholine

See "Neuromuscular blockers" on page 111.

Terbutaline

Action: Preferential β-2 adrenergic agonist; preferential effect not demonstrated clinically. Used as bronchodilator. Significant airflow improvement 15 min, peak 30-60 min after SQ administration, duration 1.5-4 hours. Elimination half-life 3 hr for most, though 6-10 hr in some patients. Unlabelled use as tocolytic.

Dose: 0.25mg SQ. May repeat in 15-30 minutes. Max 0.5mg/4hrs.

Renal failure: $T_{\frac{1}{2}}$ unknown. Use 50% GFR 10-50, avoid for GFR<10.

[213] AM Gillis, et al, "Quinidine pharmacokinetics in patients with arryhthmia: effects of left ventricular dysfunction," J Am Coll Cardiol 1995; 25(5):989-94.

[214] C Bode, et al, "Randomized comparison of coronary thrombolysis achieved with double-bolus reteplase and front-loaded, accelerated alteplase in patients with acute myocardial infarction," Circulation, 1996;94(5):891-8.

[215] "ISIS-3: a randomised comparison of streptokinase vs tPA vs anistreplase and of aspirin plus heparin vs heparin alone among 41,299 cases of suspected acute myocardial infarction," Lancet 1992;339:753.

Interactions: TCAs & MAOI potentiate sympathomimetics.
Side-effects: Hyperadrenergic state
Pregnancy: Class B.

Thiosulfate

See "Overdosage" section under "Nitroprusside" on page 113.

Tissue Plasminogen Activator (tPA)

Action: Converts plasminogen to plasmin which degrades fibrin clots. Higher affinity for fibrin-bound plasminogen than to produce less generalized "lytic state;" effect probably not clinically significant. Recombinant human product has less potential for allergic reactions. Short T½ thought to speed reperfusion. Reduces mortality & preserves LV function in acute MI, modestly superior to other thrombolytics[216]. Used also in hemodynamically unstable pulmonary emboli, and in acute arterial thromboembolism. Used early in acute ischemic stroke

Kinetics: Half-life 5-8 min, prolonged in liver failure.

Contraindications: **Absolute:** Active bleeding, stroke or intracranial/spinal surgery in past 2 months, intracranial neoplasm, suspected aortic dissection. **Relative:** Previous puncture of noncompressible vessels; surgery, organ biopsy in past 10d; serious GI bleed in past 10d-3mo; serious trauma or CPR in past 10d; diabetic proliferative retinopathy; anticoagulation; severe liver & renal disease; uncontrolled HTN > 180/110; high likelihood of intracardiac thrombus, eg MS/Afib; bacterial endocarditis; pregnancy/postpartum 10d; active menstruation.

IV: **Acute MI:** Front-loaded "GUSTO" regimen: 15 mg IV bolus followed by 0.75 mg/kg infusion over 30 min (maximum 50 mg) and then 0.50 mg/kg over 60 min (maximum 35 mg). Combine with IV heparin 5000 u bolus then 1000u/hr infusion adjusted to keep aPTT>60s over 48hr. Give within 6-24 hrs of pain onset[217]. **PE** (with hemodynamic compromise or involvement of ≥ an entire lobe): 100 mg infusion over 2 hours followed by standard heparin therapy after aPTT returns to twice normal. **Stroke**[218]: Selection: Ischemic stroke onset within 180 min, CT scan demonstrating no intracranial hemorrhage. Exclusion: No trauma or stroke in past 3 mo, SBP>185 or DBP>110 after "nonaggressive" BP tx (topical NTG, labetalol to 20 mg IV), seizure at onset of stroke, glucose > 400 mg/dL, coagulopathy, others as for MI. IV: 0.9 mg/kg up to 90 mg given as 10% bolus and 90% infused over 60 min. No anticoagulants or antiplatelet drugs × 24°. Outcome: Pts randomized to tPA vs placebo more likely to have favorable 3-mo outcome (eg 44% vs 32% Glasgow outcome scale≤1), but more likely to have symptomatic intracranial hemorrhage (6.4% vs 0.6%). No significant mortality effect or 24° neurologic improvement.

Adverse reactions: Hemorrhage (see above), reperfusion arrhythmias.

Reversal[219] for hemorrhage: FFP, cryoprecipitate, ε-aminocaproic acid.

Triiodothyronine (T3)

Action: Thyroid hormone. Acts directly unlike thyroxine (T4), a prodrug which requires peripheral conversion to T3 for action. Shorter T½~1d, compared to ~7d for T4. Rapidly increases metabolic activity in hypothyroidism, may precipitate myocardial ischemia or infarction (note ↑ cholesterol from hypothyroidism accelerates coronary disease). Not commercially available IV.

Indication: T3 is generally avoided except in life-threatening hypothyroidism in which

[216] GUSTO investigators, "The effects of tissue-plasminogen activator, streptokinase, or both on coronary-artery patency, ventricular function, and survival after acute myocardial infarction," N Engl J Med 1993; 329:1615.

[217] "ISIS-3: a randomised comparison of streptokinase vs tPA vs anistreplase and of aspirin plus heparin vs heparin alone among 41,299 cases of suspected acute myocardial infarction," Lancet 339:753, 1992.

[218] NINDS investigators, "Tissue plasminogen activator for acute ischemic stroke," N Engl J Med. 1995;333(24):1581-7.

[219] Sane DC, et al, "Bleeding during thrombolytic therapy for acute myocardial infarction: mechanisms and management," Ann Intern Med 1989;111(12):1010-22.

(1) T4 monotherapy would pose unacceptably delay in recovery, or (2) Concurrent severe nonthyroidal illness inhibits peripheral conversion from T4 to T3, rendering thyroxine administration futile.

PO: 25µg po/NG q 6 hr until response, then switch to thyroxine.
IV[220]: Mix L-T3 in 0.1 N NaOH to concentration of 250 µg/mL. Dilute 10-fold in NS + 2% albumin to final concentration 25µg/mL. Store < 1 wk at 4°C protected from light. Dose same as po.

Vasopressin

Action: Antidiuretic hormone, potent direct vasoconstrictor independent of adrenergic mechanisms, procoagulant . Used in esophageal varix hemorrhage to reduce portal pressure, hepatic flow, and as procoagulant. Used also in diabetes insipidus, as GI promotility agent, and as vasopressor.

Kinetics: Hepatic and renal metabolism. T½10-20 min.
IV: **UGI hemorrhage:** 0.1-0.6 U/min. Mix 100U/100mL D5 at 6mL/hr=0.1U/min. Combine with NTG 40-400µg/min. DI: 5-10U SQ q 8-12h.

Side effect: Myocardial ischemia via coronary vasoconstriction, SIADH or water intoxication, abd cramps, skin necrosis if exsanguinated, sweating.

Interactions: Ganglionic blocking agents markedly increase vasopressor effects. Antidiuretic effect potentiated by carbamazepine, TCAs, clofibrate, fludrocortisone, chlorpropamide. Antidiuretic effect antagonized by norepinephrine, lithium, alcohol, demeclocycline.

Vecuronium

See "Neuromuscular blockers" on page 111.

Verapamil[221]

Action: Slow-calcium-channel antagonist. Depresses SA node, slows AV node conduction not AV bypass tracts. Exacerbates LV dysfunction. Smooth muscle relaxant causes hypotension and constipation. Used IV to interrupt reentrant rhythms involving AV node and to slow ventricular response to atrial fibrillation & flutter. Used po to lower BP, suppress angina and SVT.

Kinetics: Onset 3-5 min, liver metabolism. T½ 2 hrs acute, 4-12 hrs chronic.
IV: 0.038-0.15 mg/kg (2.5-10 mg) over 2-3 min, may repeat in 15-30 min. May infuse[222] 0.005 mg/min (typically 5-10 mg/hr) for rate control. Hypotension often responds to IV CaCl₂ (5-10 mL of 10%) over 5 min. Some physicians pretreat with IV calcium[223].

Renal failure: No adjustment; Liver failure: Reduce up to 50%.
Contraindications: Undiagnosed wide-complex tachycardia, Wolf-Parkinson-White, severe LV dysfunction, sinus node dysfunction

Adverse reactions: Hypotension, bradycardia, even asystole given IV, esp with concurrent β- blockers, digoxin, hypokalemia, or in sinus node dysfunction. Exacerbates CHF.

Interactions: Digoxin clearance halved (reduce dig dose 50%). Lithium interaction variable; carbamazepine, theophylline, cyclosporine levels increased; neuromuscular blockers potentiated; dantrolene reports of vascular collapse; cimetidine prolongs verapamil half-life.

Pregnancy: Category C.

[220] RE Weiss & S Refeluff "Hypothyroidism, nonthyroidal illness, and myxedema coma," in JB Hall, GA Schmidt, L Wood (eds) Principles of Critical Care, NY:McGraw-Hill, 1990.
[221] Zachariah PK, Sheps SG, "Verapamil," in Messerli FH (ed.) Cardiovascular Drug Therapy, Philadelphia : Saunders, 1990.
[222] Barbarash RA, et al, "Verapamil infusions in the treatment of atrial tachyarrhythmias," Crit Care Med, 1986;14(10):886-8. Iberti TJ, et al, "Use of constant-infusion verapamil for the treatment of postoperative supraventricular tachycardia," Crit Care Med, 1986;14(4):283-4.
[223] Haft JI; Habbab MA, "Treatment of atrial arrhythmias. Effectiveness of verapamil when preceded by calcium infusion," Arch Intern Med, 1986;146(6):1085-9.

Warfarin *(Coumadin)*

<u>Action</u>: Anticoagulant, blocks vitamin-K-dependent transglutamylation of factors II, VII, IX, X, C, & S. Heterogeneous half-lives of clotting factors may cause transient hypercoagulability upon starting therapy, especially in partial factor C & S deficiency. Concomitant heparin for first 48° may overcome this phenomenon.

<u>Kinetics</u>:   Hepatic metabolism, enterohepatic circulation, albumin-bound. Half-life 36 hrs, biological effect 2-5d.

<u>Adverse effects</u>: Hemorrhage, skin-necrosis, procoagulant (see above).

<u>PO</u>: 10 mg qd x 2-3d then 2.5-10 mg/d for target PT or INR.

$$INR = \left[\frac{Patient\ PT}{Control\ PT} \right]^{ISI}$$

<u>Therapeutic endpoint</u>: International Normalized Ratio (INR).[204]
The "ISI" varies with batch of reagent. For DVT prophylaxis/treatment, stroke prevention in acute MI, thromboembolism prevention in atrial fibrillation, INR 2.0-3.0. For mechanical heart valves: INR 2.5-3.5. Combination with aspirin may have incremental value[206]. Probably not warranted after coronary stenting[206]. For antiphospholipid antibody syndrome: INR > 3.0[207]. Low dose warfarin (INR 1.2-1.5) combined with aspirin less efficacious in atrial fibrillation[208].

<u>Renal failure</u>: No adjustment.

<u>Reversal</u>: INR<6.0 and no bleeding, hold drug. INR 6.0-10.0 and no bleeding or elective surgery, vitamin K 0.5-1.0 mg SQ/IV will ↓ INR in 8 hrs and expect INR 2.0-3.0 within 24hr. Repeat vitamin K pm @ 24hr. High INR without bleeding: vitamin K 2.0-3.0 mg (for INR 10-20) or 10mg (INR>20). For life-threatening bleeding, use plasma + vitamin K.

<u>Interactions</u>:   **Prolongs PT**: [amiodarone, cimetidine, disulfiram, metronidazole, omeprazole, TMP/SMX, disulfiram]:inhibit clearance, cephalosporins 2&3:vitK, thyroxine:↑ metabolism; anabolic steroids, erythromycin. **Reduces PT**: [barbiturates, carbamazepine, griseofulvin, rifampin]:↑ clearance, cholestyramine:↓ absorption, moricizine.

<u>Side effect</u>: Skin necrosis: thrombosis of venules & capillaries of SQ fat. Usually seen in protein C & S deficiency on 3rd-8th day of therapy.

<u>Pregnancy</u>: Teratogen contraindicated in first trimester. Safe to nurse.

General Drug References

Physicians' Desk Reference, 50th ed., Montvale, NJ: Medical Economics Data, 1996.

Drug Evaluations, 6th Edition, Chicago: AMA Publications, 1986.

Bennet WM et al, Drug prescribing in renal failure: dosing guidlines for adults, 3rd ed. Phildelphia: American College of Physicians, 1994.

Goldfrank, LR, Toxicologic Emergencies, 5th ed., Norwalk, CT:Appleton-Lange, 1994.

Hardman JG, et al, Goodman and Gilman's Pharmacological basis of therepeutics, 9th ed., New York: McGraw-Hill, 1996.

Messerli FH, Cardiovascular drug therapy, 2nd ed., Philadelphia: WB Saunders, 1996.

---

204 Hirsh J, et al, "Oral anticoagulants. Mechanism of action, clinical effectiveness, and optimal therapeutic range," Chest, 1995;108(4 Suppl):231S-246S.

205 Turpie AG, et al, "A comparison of aspirin with placebo in patients treated with warfarin after heart-valve replacement," N Engl J Med, 1993;329(8):524-9.

206 Schomig A, et al, "A randomized comparison of antiplatelet and anticoagulant therapy after the placement of coronary-artery stents," N Engl J Med, 1996;334(17):1084-9.

207 Khamashta MA, et al, "The management of thrombosis in the antiphospholipid-antibody syndrome," N Engl J Med, 1995;332(15):993-7.

208 "Adjusted-dose warfarin versus low-intensity, fixed-dose warfarin plus aspirin for high-isk patients with atrial fibrillation: Stroke prevention in atrial fibrillation III randomised clinical trial, Lancet 1996; 348:633-638.

Index